MW01014293

JOHN ABEL
QUENTIN ABRAHANTE
JEANNE ACHENBACH
LISA ADALI
PAMELA ADAMS
MONICA ADDUCI
SARAH AESCHLEMAN
JOAN AGINS
RAMIRO AGUERO
EMMA AGUERO
JEANNINE ALAMEDA
KIM ALBERT
JOHN ALEXANDER
AKBAR ALINANI
REY ALMARIO
CAROLYN ALTEMOSE
ALAN ALTEMOSE
CARL ANDERSON
ERIC ANDERSON
ROBERT ANGELI
DAVID ANGELL
CRAIG ANGLEMIRE
DAMON ANTHONY
NORMA APONTE
JOHN ARANCIO
MARY ARGOT
DIANE ARISTARCO
JATINDER ARORA
HARI ASTHANA
PHILIP ATTEBERRY
MARIAN AUGUSTUS
ROBIN AUTH
WILLIAM AVERBECK
J. SCOTT BAILEY
RONALD BAIR
JOHN BAIRD
ANDREA BAKER
MICHAEL BALLEW
MARY BALUTA
CAROLYN BAMERT
AMY BAPTISTE
JAY BARBER
DONALD BARI
LORRAINE BARKER
KAREN BARNES
KRISTEN BARRADALE
KELLY BARTLETT
RICHARD BARTLEWSKI
SHIREEN BASHIR
SHEILA BASSETT
ROBERT BATES
MICHAEL BAWDUNIAK
HEATHER BEATTIE
RONALD BEAVERS
ROBERT BECKER
CAROLYN BECKER
ROBERT BELOW
LINDA BENDER
DEANNA BENSON
LISA BENTLER

CHRISTINE BENTON
STACY BERECEK
JOHN BERKLEY
ARNOLD BERRY
PETA-LYNN BESECKER
CHERYL BEVAN
MARTHA BICKEL
LAURA BINCAROWSKY
GERALD BINGHAM
JILL BIRTWELL
KAREN BISCARDI
JENNIFER BISHER
BARBARA BITTNER
A. MICHAEL BLOH
JENNIFER BLUM
PAMELA BLUST
GERALD BONE
IRENE BONIFACE
SHAWN BOOKHOUT
TIMOTHY BOOTH
WILLIAM BORER
SANDRA BOWEN
ROGER BOWMAN
BRUCE BOWMAN
RENEE BOYD
DAMIAN BRAGA
PATRICIA BRAUN
SCOTT BRAY
DAMON BRESHEARS
KENNETH BRIGHAM
RICHARD BRINLEY
LAURIE BROST
RANDALL BROWN
JAMES BROWN
BETH BROWN
RALEIGH BROWN
ANITA BROWN
SAMUEL BROWN
DOUGLAS BROWN
MARY BROWN
GERALD BRUNS
CAROL BRYAN
STEPHANIE BULS
BERNADINE BURCH
LINDA BURGOS
JUDY BURKE
JENNIFER BURRIER
KATHLEEN BUSH
EVELYN BUTTS
MICHAEL BYBEL
JAMES BYRNE
GARY CALANDRA
MARY CALLEN
JOHN CAMAEREI
GORDON CAMPBELL
SEAN CAMPBELL
CYNTHIA CAMPO
KURT CANNON
MICHAEL CANTREL
FRED CAPILUPO

CYNTHIA CAPILUPO
CHRISTINE CAPONIGRO
AARON CAPORUSCIO
BARBARA CAPRIOLI
PATRICK CARANGELO
DONALD CARAVELLO
MONICA CARBONE
STEVEN CARTER
KATHLEEN CARTRIGHT
DANIEL CASEY
ANDREA CASSADY
LEE CASTAGNOS
TYLER CASTOR
JAMES CAWLEY
NORMAN CEASE
JENNIFER CERENE
DEANA CERRA
PRADIP CHAKRAVARTY
CYNTHIA CHAPMAN
ADITYA CHAUDHARY
ROBERT CHECK
ROBIN CHEW
MARIA CHILLE
GREGG CHRISTIANSON
PATRICIA CIAFREI
MARTIN CITROLA
TIMOTHY CLEARY
MONIQUE CLEVERLEY
DAVID COBB
BERNARD COBLE
ALLEN COFFMAN
CHRISTINE COGLISER
LUCY COHOWICZ
ANTHONY COLELLO
MICHAEL COLEMAN
JOHN COLLINS
THERESA COLTON
JAMES COMMODORE
GAYLE CONDON
RONALD CONLEY
ADRIENNE CONLIN
PHILIP CONNOR
CYNTHIA COOK
GRACE COOPER
ANGELA CORONA
TODD COSSICK
WILLARD COSTANZO
STEPHEN COTTON
LISA COURTADE
DOUGLAS COVENEY
SARAH COX
TAMI-ANN COX
TODD COYNE
JOANNE CREAMER
MELANY CREEL
RYAN CROSS
CECELIA CROWE
ROSSANA CUELLAR
DENNIS CULLEN
JAMES CUMINS

TIMOTHY CUNNIFF
JEFFREY CURTIS
BRIAN CUSTARD
CHERYL CUSTARD
WILLIAM CWYK
SUSAN CZUPRYNA
KATHLEEN D'ANDREA
RICHARD DABNER
GERALD DAHLING
ZHONGDONG DAI
BRUCE DAMBOISE
DONNA DAVIS
MICHELLE DAVIS
BRUCE DAVIS
GERALD DAVITT
WENDY DE HAVEN
AUGUSTINE DE SANTIS
HELEN DE SORDI
BARBARA DEAN
SUSAN DECARO
DAVID DECKER
CHRISTOPHER DECKER
DENISE DECKER
JANET DEGRAW
DAVID DEITZER
GAIL DETRICK
ELIZABETH DEWITSKY
CINDY DI IOIA
TINA DIECKMANN
MARK DIEHL
RHONDA DIEHL
ROSEMARY DIETRICH
JOSEPH DIMATTIO
RICHARD DIPAOLO
CAROLYN DITTUS
DAWN DOGGETT
MOLLY DOLAN
DONNA DOLL
JOHN DONSCHIETZ
DAVID DORAN
LORRAINE DOYLE
JANET DOZOIS
GAIL DRAKE
EDWARD DRAKE
ANDREA DREISBACH
COLLEEN DUCAS
MICHAEL DUCAS
DIANE DUDICK
CYNTHIA DUKES
F. SCOTT DUNCAN
MICHAEL DUNN
MARIA DURAND
D. ALEX DWOSKIN
PATRICIA DYSON
KATHLEEN DYSON
LORI EASTERDAY
BRENT EATON
GARY EBBERT
KIRK EDWARDS
HELEN EILBER

ROBERT EILER	DENISE GAUGHAN	BEN HARRISON	LAURA JODZ
LILLIAN ELDERS	ALAN GELFAND	BRUCE HARTLEY	KATHALEEN JOFFE
CAROL ELLIS	JAMES GEORGE	JEAN HARTMAN	FRANKLIN JOHN
THERESA ELLIS	PETER GERARD	PATRICIA HARVEY	MARK JOHNSON
FRANK EPIFANO	CELESTINE GESKEY	PAMELA HASARA	JAYNE JOHNSON
LORNE ERDILE	KARISSA GETTINGS	JOAN HAWK	ROBIN JOHNSON
JENNIFER ERICKSON	SUSAN GETZ	DENISE HEASTER	DAVID JOHNSON
RYAN ESCO	KRISTINA GILLIES	WILLIAM HEASTER	SCOTT JOHNSON
PATRICIA ESCOBAR	CHRISTINE GILLIS	ERIC HEDGE	AMY JOHNSTON
FRED ESCOBAR	JOSEPH GIUMENTO	ANGELA HEH	DONALD JOHNSTON
RICHARD EVANS	KERRY GO	MARTHA HEISE	ROBERT JONES
KAYLA EVARTS	AMBER GODFREY	DANIEL HEIST	ERIC JONES
RICKIE EVERETT	GREGORY GOFFREDA	MAUREEN HELD	CARMELA KAHN
TRACY FAHR	DONNA GOLASZEWSKI	RONALD HELLER	MICHAEL KARETA
THOMAS FAHRNER	PHILLIP GOMEZ	KIM HENDERSON	JENNIFER KASZTEJNA
LEONARD FAIRFIELD	BRUCE GONTZ	SANDRA HENRY	SANFORD KAUFMAN
ROBERT FAIRSERVICE	KAREN GONZALEZ	ANDRIA HERNANDEZ	KIMBERLY KAUNITZ
MELISSA FARNHAM	LILLIAN GONZALEZ	DIANE HERRMANN	SUSANNE KAVITSKI
KEVIN FARRELL	JUDITH GOODE	MARK HERRON	COLLEEN KEATING
WILLIAM FARRELL	JOHN GOODREAU	SHERILYN HERRON	DARIN KELLY
TRACIE FARRY	DAVID GOTTLIEB	KENNETH HERRON	MICHAEL KIELAR
SHARON FAUST	VALENTINA GOUMAKOS	JEFFREY HESTER	ROBERT KIERES
WILLIAM FELL	DEBORAH GOWER	JANE HILLOCK	BRUCE KILBY
CHRISTOPHER FENN	CHRISTY GRADY	JAMES HINTON	GAIL KILBY
IRENE FENNELL	CHRISTINE GRANT	THOMAS HODAR	DAESEONG KIM
GARY FENNELL	GREGORY GRASS	TERESA HOEHNE	CHARLES KIMMEL
DEBORAH FERENCAK	JOHN GRAU	HEATHER HOFFMANN	ROSEMARY KINDREW
LAURA FERGUSON	ELEANOR GRAVEL	WILLIAM HOFFNER	JENNIFER KINSLEY
CHRISTOPHER FERNER	MARYANN GRAY	MARK HOLDEMAN	CHRISTOPHER KIRALY
TODD FERRANTI	KAREN GRAY	MARK HOLMAN	HEIDI KIRALY
LISA FETTERS	JOSEFINA GREEN	JOHN HOLT	CHRISTINE KIRBY
RONALD FILIPSKI	PATRICIA GREENE	STEPHEN HOLTON	RUDOLPH KIRCHER
BRIAN FINLAYSON	CAROLYN GREGOIRE	KIMBERLY HOOK	PAUL KIRKCONNELL
NANCY FINNERTY	ROLAND GRISSOM	CHRISTOPHER HOOPES	DOUGLAS KIRKMAN
JENNIFER FISCHER	MARGARET GROTLE	CHAD HOOVER	KIMBERLY KIRSCH
RAYMOND FISHER	CONNIE GROVER	MARY HOPKINS	KIMBERLY KIZER
EILEEN FLAHERTY	MICHAEL GRUETZMACHER	JOANNE HORN	KELLEE JO KLEINTOP
WILLIAM FLOUNDERS	BADMAKA GRUM	JASON HORN	JEFF KLEINTOP
CINDY FLUEGEL	JAMES GUARDINO	PHILIP HOSBACH	RENA KLEPACKI
REGINA FLUEGEL	KENNETH GUITO	TIMOTHY HOWE	ROBERT KLEPADLO
ARTHUR FOOSE	PATRICK GUTE	WILLIAM HOWENSTINE	KEITH KLINE
SHIRLEY FRANCIS	SANDY GUTTING	MATTHEW HUDSON	LAURA KNECHT
DEBORAH FRANCIS	JEFFREY HACKMAN	ROBERT HUEBNER	STEPHEN KNOPF
DIANE FRANCIS	WILLIAM HAGAN	KRISTINE HUNT	ERNEST KNOX
JAMES FRANKS	PATSY HAGERMAN	KEVIN HUSS	NANETTE KOEHN
SUONG FRANKS	FREDERICK HAHN	AILEEN HYDE	BARBARA KOLCZ
SAMUEL FRANTZ	JONATHAN HAINES	DEBRA HYNOSKI	ALEXANDER KONOPKA
CHERYLYNN FRANTZ	PETER HALASZ	ERIC IGNATIN	ROBERT KORAB
E MICHAEL FREIN	SCOTT HALLAM	CARL IRVIN	EDWARD KOTHERA
JAMES FROESCHLE	ALMA HALSTEAD	KIMBERLY JACKSON	JOHN KOZEL
LESLIE FUCHS	RANDY HALSTEAD	SHARON JACQUES	KATHLEEN KRAIG-DI IOIA
DEBRA FULMER	LEO HALSTEAD	ROBERTA JAMES	MONTE KRAMER
WILLIAM FULTON	DAWN HAMBLIN	SHIRLEY JAMES	PATRICK KRESGE
BARBARA FURNARI	MARK HANKINS	WALTER JAMES	ROBERT KROGMEIER
JERRY GAIGE	PETER HANSCOME	NICOLE JAYCOX	JEANNE KRON
JOHN GALLAGHER	JANICE HANSCOME	PATRICIA JEAN JEAN	JOSEPH KRUK
LINDA GALLAGHER	BRENDA HANVEY	JOSEPH JELLOCK	LINDA KRUMMELL
MICHAEL GARUD	MAURICE HARMON	SABRA JENKINS	PATRICIA KRUSE
AMY GARY	LINDA HARMS	JENNIFER JENNINGS	ALEX KUCERA
JOHN GASPER	ARTHUR HARRIS	ELIZABETH JIMENEZ	AARON KUNDIN

The Spirit of Swiftwater

100 Years at the Pocono Labs

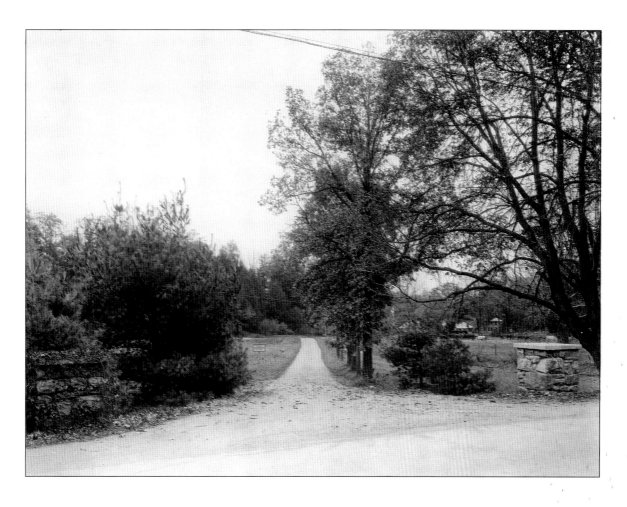

JEFF WIDMER

SCRANTON: UNIVERSITY OF SCRANTON PRESS

Contents

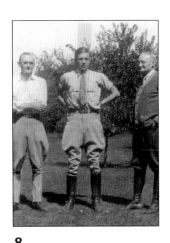

8

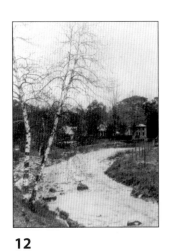

12

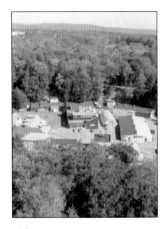

68

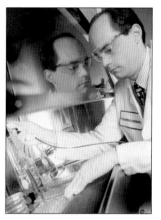

102

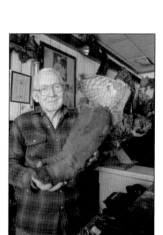

118

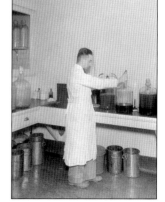

144

© 1998 by the University of Scranton Press

All Rights Reserved

Library of Congress Cataloging-in-Publication Data

Widmer, Jeff.
    The spirit of swiftwater: 100 years at the Pocono labs/
Jeff Widmer.
      p.   cm.
    Includes index.
    ISBN 0-940866-74-9
    1. Smallpox vaccine–Pennsylvania–History. 2. Slee, Richard M.,
1867-1945. 3. Vaccines industry–Pennsylvania–History. 4. Pocono
Biological Laboratories (Swiftwater, Pa.)–History I. Title.
QR189.5.S6W53   1998
614.5'21–dc21   98-40902
                                               CIP

Distribution

University of Toronto Press

2250 Military Road

Tonawanda NY 14150

PRINTED IN THE UNITED STATES OF AMERICA

Being part of Pasteur Mérieux Connaught gives us the largest critical mass for developing and marketing products throughout the world.

— Dave Williams
President and Chief Operating Officer
Pasteur Mérieux Connaught USA

Acknowledgments

*T*his book would not have been possible without the cooperation and contributions of senior management and the employees of Pasteur Mérieux Connaught. I am indebted to various individuals as well. Willard Webster wrote several detailed histories of the early years of the laboratories. Damian Braga and Gary Ebbert spent hours shaping the final section of the book. Dr. Don Metzgar allowed me to quote freely from *Metzgar's Unofficial History and Commentary*. His tour of the current Swiftwater facility that sunny day in July 1996 was very

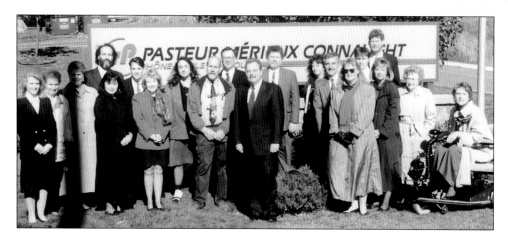

instructive. From the "hellos" and hugs he received, it is evident that, even in retirement, he is still widely known and respected within the company.

I would like to thank Dr. Ralph Vosdingh and the members of the Swiftwater Historical Society: Mary Lynn Argot, Barbara Bittner, Randy Brown, Gerry Bruns, Susan Getz, Jake Keiper, Chris Kirby, Junior Leauber, Mike Macerollo, Don Metzgar, Susan Polizzotto, Kathy Rose, Ricky Smith, Tom Thorn, Clair Wallingford, and Rodney Waltz.

Thanks to Catherine Newberry for initiating the history-book project and to Chris Kirby and the members of the book's Editorial Board — Mary Lynn Argot, Damian Braga, Len Fairfield, Aileen Hyde, Len Lavenda, Colleen Ducas, Don Metzgar, and Ralph Vosdingh.

Jo Seale in Human Resources provided editorial support. Rodney Waltz and Mike Macerollo, the keepers of the keys to the archive room, lugged and hauled boxes for 2 weeks while I dug through a century of papers. Clair Wallingford has preserved not only paper but original equipment for posterity. It is through their contribution and others that Swiftwater's artifacts will be preserved.

Thanks to the staff at the Eastern Monroe Public Library — Phil Hearne, Barbara Keiser, and Ann Kane — and Janet Mishkin of the Monroe County Historical Society for their help in locating records and people. Thanks also go to the people who so graciously gave of their time for interviews: Georges Hibon, Dave Williams, Damian Braga, Gary Ebbert, Phil Hosbach, Walter Woods, Mary Lynn Argot, attorney Alex "Buzz" Bensinger, Dr. Don Metzgar, G. Willard Webster, Dr. Anthony Bolyn, Alun Davies, Peter Campbell, Doug Reynolds, Jean-Jacques Bertrand, Dr. Ralph Vosdingh, Barbara Bittner, Clair Wallingford, Ellen Regan, Dr. Howard Six, Sy Katz, and Jessie Eisel.

Thanks go to Keith Nealy and David Coulter for providing much of the contemporary photography for the book.

Many others provided support and pointed to additional sources of information: Pam Spears, Bill Farrell, Chris Grant, Kathy Rector, attorney Jeffrey Wright, Lorraine Doyle, John Appel, Bill Clark, Brian McKenna, Jack E. Termine at the Medical Research Library of Brooklyn, Mariam Touba of the New York Historical Society, and Barbara Slee Diefenderfer, wife of the late Arthur Slee.

Finally, a special thanks goes to the great-grandchildren of Dr. Richard Slee, Prescott Slee and his sister, Deborah Slee Gibbs, for rummaging through attics, furnishing photographs, and copying pages from the family Bible. They have supplied valuable information about a man whose accomplishments otherwise may have been lost.

Jeff Widmer
Swiftwater, Pennsylvania
August 1997

Left: Employees and management at Pasteur Mérieux Connaught observe the company's name change in 1996.

Below: Packaging from Dr. Richard Slee's smallpox vaccine product.

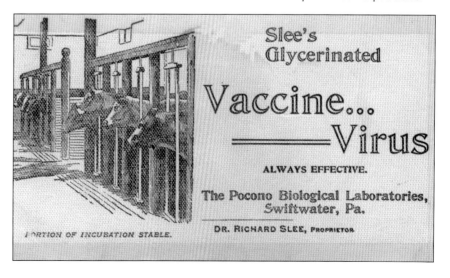

Slee's Glycerinated Vaccine... ===Virus

ALWAYS EFFECTIVE.

The Pocono Biological Laboratories, Swiftwater, Pa.

DR. RICHARD SLEE, PROPRIETOR

PORTION OF INCUBATION STABLE.

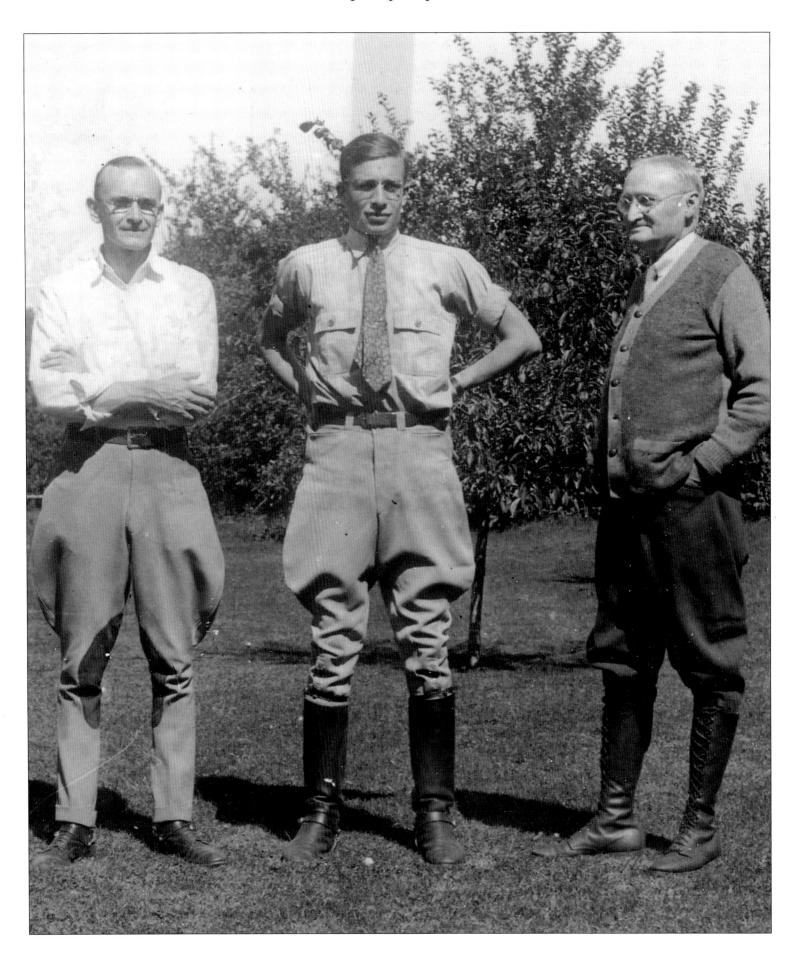

Preface

The foundation of the laboratories had all of the elements of the American free-enterprise system — ambition, tragedy, failure, and success.

— G. Willard Webster

*W*e take vaccines for granted. We get our shots as kids and forget about the process until we have children of our own. In the Western Hemisphere, we generally don't see the diseases that plague the Third World. We call them preventable.

A hundred years ago, the science of immunology was struggling, and so were its advocates. Just before the founder of the Swiftwater Laboratories, Dr. Richard Slee, was born in 1867, the French biologist Louis Pasteur had proven the germ theory of disease. It wasn't until 1885 that Pasteur field tested his vaccine for rabies. Twelve years later, when Slee built his laboratory to manufacture smallpox vaccine in Swiftwater, Pennsylvania, the disease was still considered a major threat to public health. It would not be eradicated worldwide until 1980. To make matters worse, the technology of the time caused more problems than it solved in many people. Because of adverse reactions, vaccines of the time stimulated fear as well as immunity.

There were other obstacles. From currency panic to gold rush, the ups and downs of the American economy challenged even the heartiest entrepreneur. Wars provided both opportunity and pain. The industrial boom came of age. The nation expanded. During his 40 years in business, Slee would struggle financially, closing the Swiftwater Labs in 1908, reopening them 3 years later, and finally selling them to the National Drug Co. in 1930. To raise capital, he took on a partner and moonlighted with state health agencies in Pennsylvania and New York. As for his company, it would go through numerous ownership changes and totter on the brink of ruin before emerging today as Pasteur Mérieux Connaught, a global leader in human vaccines.

Despite a century of change, the Swiftwater Labs have always faced the same challenges — funding research, finding distributors, managing liability, beating competition. While the business has grown from five people in the early 1900s

Facing page: Three generations of Slees. From left, Arthur, Richard E., and the founder, Dr. Richard Slee.

Below: Dr. Richard Slee in 1912.

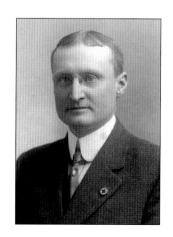

to more than a thousand people today, the challenges Slee faced at the turn of the century will continue into the next millennium. During World War I, it was a reliance on military contracts for almost all business. In the 1920s, there were distribution problems. Through the war years, the focus was on differentiating the products from those of the competition. In the 1970s, recovering from the disastrous swine flu campaign posed a challenge. In the 1980s, concentrating on positioning vaccines as an essential part of health care, not as a generic com-

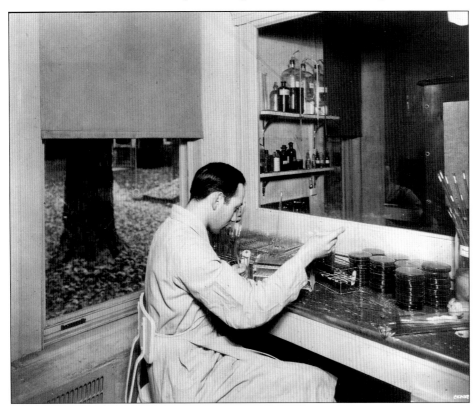

modity. In the 1990s, the challenge comes from a global marketplace and the competition it creates.

Throughout four wars and six changes in ownership, the people of Swiftwater have responded to those challenges with resourcefulness and innovation. They have built the company from the ground up on three occasions. They have turned a profit even during the most challenging times. They have practiced good science in the face of uncertainty, developing vaccines that will keep millions of children and adults healthy for generations to come.

The job isn't over. According to the World Health Organization (WHO) and the United Nations Children's Fund, more than 12 million children under age 5 die every year; as many as 2 million of those deaths result from diseases that could be prevented by vaccines offered through WHO's Expanded Programme on Immunization. "While the war against polio is being won," WHO reported in 1996, "the battle against other vaccine-preventable diseases has a long way to run. In 1994, over a million children died from measles, almost 500,000 from neonatal tetanus, and almost 400,000 from whooping cough."

In the United States, a million children are still not immunized at the age-appropriate time, and some 5,000 contract whooping cough each year.

From the beginning, Dr. Slee's small company had ties to the rest of the world. In 1896, with the aid of the smallpox formula he received from the

Pasteur Institute, Slee began turning his wife's property on the east side of what is now Route 611 into the Pocono Biological Laboratories. Similar events were happening overseas. The following year, Marcel Mérieux, after studying under Pasteur at the Pasteur Institute, founded Institut Biologique Mérieux. For years, Slee and Mérieux operated independently of one another. After the First World War, Mérieux set up a new laboratory at Marcy l'Etoile near Lyon, France. Slee left the business in 1927 when he leased, and later sold, his laboratories to the National Drug Co., but the company lived on under various owners. In 1978, the Canadian firm Connaught Laboratories Ltd. purchased the facility Slee had created and named it Connaught Laboratories Inc. In 1985, Pasteur Institute's commercial vaccine operations were united with Mérieux under the name Pasteur Mérieux Serums & Vaccins. Four years later, PMsv completed the circle that began in the early 1890s with Dr. Slee's visit to France by purchasing the Canadian and Swiftwater operations. In November 1996, the company began doing business as Pasteur Mérieux Connaught.

Over the course of a century, the Swiftwater facility has weathered depression and neglect. It has overcome problems of liability and finance. Through wars and mergers, prosperity and peace, it has reinvented itself to become a multi-million-dollar business with world-class partners and a global reach. What began as a few stone buildings and a stable has become an innovative company that brings health and hope to millions — the direct result of the indomitable spirit of its staff.

Here's to the next 100 years.

Facing page: The Swiftwater Labs in 1932.

Below: Connaught brochure from 1993.

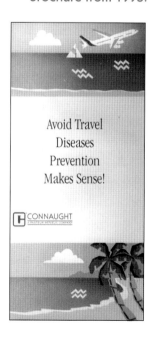

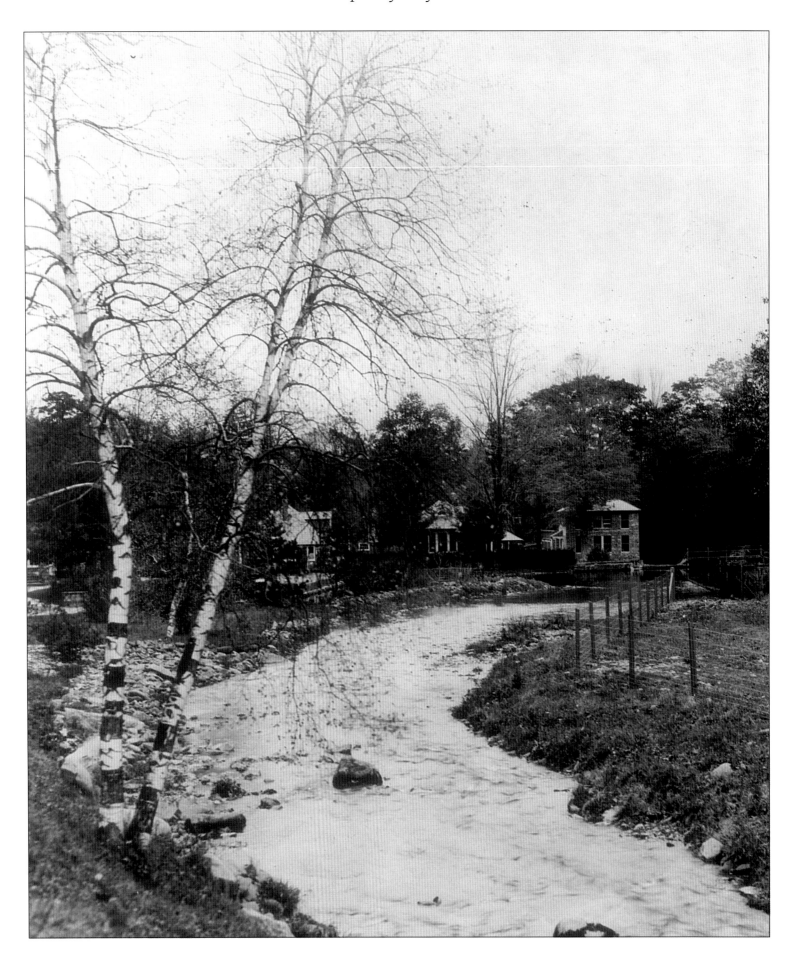

Birth of an Industry

If Dr. Slee had outlined a plan and then placed his requirements into the hands of Nature for fulfillment, he could not have been directed to a location better adapted to his needs.

— *Times-Democrat*, Stroudsburg, Pennsylvania, 1915

American Enterprise (1865–95)

*I*t was the golden age of American industry. In 1867, the year Richard M. Slee was born, Russia sold Alaska to the United States and the first transcontinental railroad was completed. Over the next 20 years, John D. Rockefeller would found Standard Oil. Louis Pasteur would prove it possible to protect humans from disease through vaccination. In New York City, Thomas Edison would build the world's first electric power plant.

Everywhere in the Western world, advances in industry and science signaled a new era of prosperity and health. In Slee's hometown of Brooklyn, N.Y., work started in 1869 on the Brooklyn Bridge, the world's longest suspension span when completed in 1883. During his early years, Slee would see George Eastman introduce the Kodak camera, Henry Ford mass produce the automobile, and Guglielmo Marconi tame radio waves. As he turned 20, Slee watched as New York unveiled the Statue of Liberty. The event would foreshadow another gift from France years later, one that would change the course of an industry.

For Americans, the years following the Civil War were a time of Manifest Destiny, an age when science and industry could conquer almost anything, from distance to disease. For a future entrepreneur with an interest in health, Richard M. Slee was born at an opportune time, on September 15, 1867. His parents had just moved from Bond Head, Canada, to the promised land of New York's biggest town. It was a time that would produce great science and great scientists: Born that year were Marie Sklodowska Curie and William Thomson, later known as Lord Kelvin. It was another geographic link that would come full-circle 100 hundred years later, when a business started by the son of a Canadian

Facing page: Birches line the Swiftwater Creek at the Slee lab, while pastures rise to the right, where Bldg. 45 now stands.

Below: Seal of Pennsylvania on letter certifying the lab in 1900.

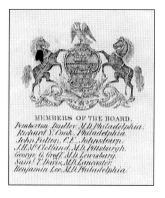

MEMBERS OF THE BOARD,
Pemberton Dudley, M.D. Philadelphia;
Richard Y. Cook, Philadelphia;
John Fulton, C.E., Johnstown;
J.H. McClelland, M.D. Pittsburgh;
George G. Groff, M.D. Lewisburg;
Sam.l T. Davis, M.D. Lancaster;
Benjamin Lee, M.D. Philadelphia.

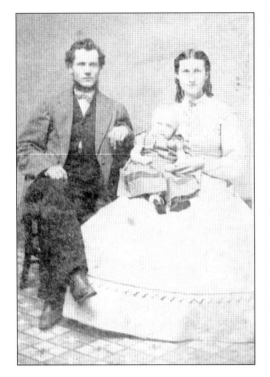

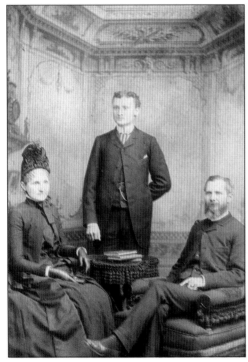

Top: Richard C. Slee
and Marie J. Slee
with their son,
Richard M., in 1868.

Above: Richard M.
with his parents,
circa 1883.

immigrant would be purchased by that country's leading producer
of vaccines.

Richard's parents, Richard Child Slee and Maria Jane Orr, had
married in 1865, then moved to Brooklyn, where Richard senior
engaged in a dry goods business. The Slees prospered with the
times. Richard's sister, Elizabeth Maria Slee, was born in 1871, followed by a brother, Alfred Hyde Slee, in 1877.

Brooklyn presented newcomers with a multitude of contrasts
and opportunities. Mansions of affluent merchants contrasted with
the tenements near the docks. The largest of five counties that
would unite to form Greater New York in 1898, Brooklyn suffered
from the challenges of a big city, including all of the health and
sanitation problems of the time. Death from what later generations
would call preventable diseases was common, and the Slee family
did not escape their wrath. A year after his birth, Alfred died of
meningitis; 5 years later, Lizzie died of scarlet fever. Richard was
11 and 16, respectively, when his brother and sister died.

There is no way of knowing how those deaths affected him, or
whether they influenced his decision to attend medical school.
But in 1891, Richard Slee graduated from the Long Island
College Hospital with a number of awards and went to work for
Dr. George M. Sternberg, a fellow bacteriologist who would have
a great impact on American medicine — through the publication
of his book, *A Manual of Bacteriology*, the first comprehensive work
on the subject in America, and later through his work as the surgeon general of the United States.

When Slee began his career, the science of immunology was in
its infancy. Pasteur had just discovered, in 1885, a vaccine for
rabies. Despite successes with immunization in the United States,
the medical community still considered smallpox a major threat.
Recorded as early as the time of Moses, it had spread like a plague
throughout the world. During the sixteenth century in Mexico, 3.5 million
people died of the disease. In nineteenth-century England, from 7% to 9% of all
deaths were attributed to smallpox.

The new science of immunology had proven vaccines could save lives. It had
progressed quickly from the late 1700s, when British physician Dr. Edward
Jenner discovered that smallpox could be prevented by inoculating people with
the substance from cowpox lesions. The vaccine worked. According to the New

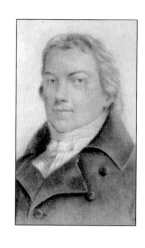

York City Health Department, the death rate from smallpox in 1869 was 21.9 per 100,000 people. In 1876, New York's Vaccination Corps fanned out to inoculate the city. The following year, the death rate per 100,000 people had dropped to 0.18.

But with vaccination came side effects that troubled the medical community and alarmed the public. Calves were used in the production of the American smallpox vaccine. The abdominal surface of the calf was shaved, the skin cleaned and scarified, and the virus rubbed over the scarified area. Five to seven days later, the area would be covered with scabs. They were removed, ground with a small amount of diluent, and sealed into glass capillary tubes, or dried on ivory points, which were then used to scrape a person's skin to administer the vaccine. Since the growth field on the calf could not be maintained in a sterile condition, bacteria of all types found their way into the final product. The vaccine would then cause infection in otherwise healthy people.

To Dr. Sternberg, the public's attitude must have seemed alarming. Here was a potential lifesaver that could fail because of social, not scientific, reasons. As the nation's newly appointed surgeon general in 1893, Sternberg wanted to vaccinate the general population. After hearing of a revolutionary vaccine developed at Pasteur Institute, Sternberg dispatched Slee to France to investigate.

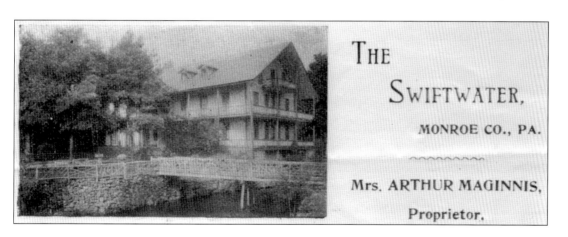

THE SWIFTWATER,

MONROE CO., PA.

Mrs. ARTHUR MAGINNIS,

Proprietor.

The report was glowing. Slee found better efficacy and fewer side effects from the French formula, which mixed the mild disinfectant glycerin with the virus to lower the bacteria count and prolong the shelf life of the vaccine — an important consideration when commercializing the product. The results so impressed Sternberg that he encouraged the young doctor to set up a private laboratory for its manufacture. Slee had already found the perfect site.

In the early 1890s, he had contracted cholera, which caused death in more than 50% of untreated cases in many parts of the world. To recuperate, he had retreated to the clean air and quiet surroundings of the Pocono Mountains in

Top: Vaccine pioneer Dr. Edward Jenner.

Left: Letterhead from the Swiftwater Inn, circa 1890.

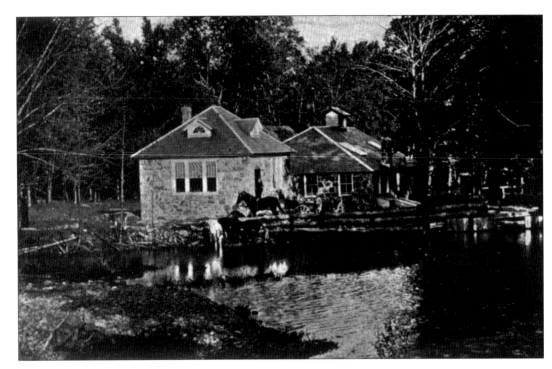

Northeast Pennsylvania, ending up at the Swiftwater Inn in the town of that name. Run by Ella and Arthur Maginnis, the property had been an original grant to Samuel Powell of Philadelphia in 1774 and now housed the couple and their daughters, one of whom was also named Ella. Born in 1870, Ella had barely reached her early twenties and must have proven quite attractive to the young doctor, who married her in 1892 and signed on as an attending physician at the inn the following year. By all accounts, it was a romance worthy of a novel. But its details were lost to history in the early 1990s when a fire at the Swiftwater Inn destroyed all remaining records.

Arthur Maginnis did not live to see his daughter's wedding. He died the year before, leaving to his widow and two grown daughters the inn, some land, and a $15,000 insurance policy.

The early 1890s were both the best and worst of times for creating a business. Monroe County bustled with resorts, the town of Delaware Water Gap, 15 miles to the southeast, holding center stage. Land that had been inhabited by the Leni Lenape and settled a century before by the British and the Dutch now sported huge hotels — the Indian Queen, the Lackawanna House, the Kittatinny House. Stroudsburg, the county seat, attracted merchants and lawyers. The railroad ran through East Stroudsburg several miles southeast of Swiftwater, and to the north in Mount Pocono, resorts, dry goods stores, and a post office signaled a thriving community. Whether by fate or good fortune, Slee had chosen the perfect site for a laboratory, with clean air, adequate roads, a ready supply of goods and labor, a pristine stream, and green pastures for the animals.

The spot may have been ideal, but the metaphoric road to it was often rocky. The nationwide Panic of 1893 plunged the business community into chaos as foreign investors withdrew capital from the U.S. economy. A severe economic

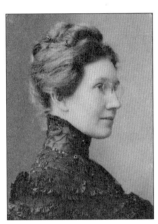

Top: Exterior of the labs in summer, as they appeared in Dr. Slee's brochure of 1903.

Above: Ella Maginnis, wife of the founder, Dr. Richard Slee.

depression raged throughout 1894, but the world, and the Slees, kept looking ahead. By the middle of the decade, Henry Ford would build his first car, Marconi would invent radio telegraphy, and Wilhelm Roentgen would discover X rays.

In Swiftwater, Arthur Maginnis Slee, the only child of Richard and Ella, was born in 1894, the year the song "The Sidewalks of New York" was written. In 1895, Louis Pasteur died. The following year, gold was discovered in the Yukon, and John Philip Sousa wrote "The Stars and Stripes Forever." The fanfare of his most famous march could only reflect the spirit of the time. Life in the United States was booming, and Richard Slee wanted to become part of that boom.

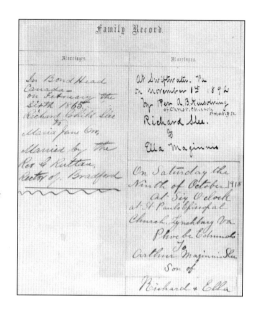

Bootstrap Science (1897–1908)

His timing was perfect. There were smallpox epidemics in Philadelphia and other cities in 1871 and 1872, and in nearby Reading in 1893 and 1894. A 1900 booklet by the Pennsylvania State Board of Health says that 1,429 cases of smallpox were reported during the statewide epidemic of 1898–1900.

Slee drafted plans for his laboratory and submitted them to the state board of health for approval in February 1897. Two months later, the plans were approved for a 4.3-acre site, left to his wife Ella by her father. On July 9, Slee constructed a laboratory that measured 37'3" by 56'4", a 2,100-square-foot structure built of local stone and native chestnut, cut on the property. He also built a frame stable for the calves that measured 31'9" by 20'6". The stable stood next to the laboratory and was connected by a covered walkway. Years later, during renovations, the keystone over the door was placed on the ground next to the original lab, now called Building 3.

Slee called his company the Pocono Biological Laboratories. Letterhead from the time lists Dr. Richard Slee as bacteriologist, and his father, Richard C. Slee, as manager, although there are no records of the elder Slee's active participation. Richard junior began producing glycerinated smallpox vaccine, which he called "vaccine virus."

Above: A page from the Slee family Bible showing record of marriages.

Left: Dr. Benjamin Lee's letter of 1900 to the labs showing they passed state inspection.

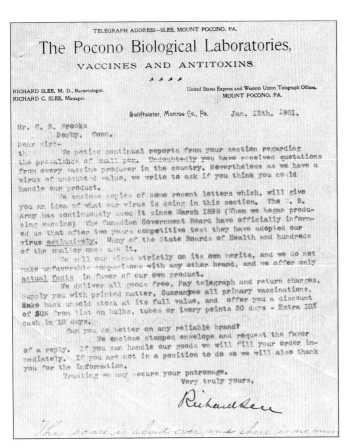

TELEGRAPH ADDRESS—SLEE, MOUNT POCONO, PA.

The Pocono Biological Laboratories,

VACCINES AND ANTITOXINS.

RICHARD SLEE, M. D., Bacteriologist.
RICHARD C. SLEE, Manager.

United States Express and Western Union Telegraph Offices,
MOUNT POCONO, PA.

Swiftwater, Monroe Co., Pa.   Jan. 12th. 1901.

Mr. C. R. Brooks
     Derby, Conn.

Dear Sir:—
     We notice continual reports from your section regarding the prevalence of small pox. Undoubtedly you have received quotations from every vaccine producer in the country. Nevertheless as we have a virus of undoubted value, we write to ask if you think you could handle our product.
     We enclose copies of some recent letters which, will give you an idea of what our virus is doing in this section. The U. S. Army has continually used it since March 1898 (When we began producing vaccine) The Canadian Government Board have officially informed us that after two years competitive test they have adopted our virus exclusively. Many of the State Boards of Health and hundreds of the smaller ones use it.
     We sell our virus strictly on its own merits, and we do not make unfavorable comparisons with any other brand, and we offer only actual facts in favor of our own product.
     We deliver all goods free, Pay telegraph and return charges, Supply you with printed matter, Guarantee all primary vaccinations, Take back unsold stock at its full value, and offer you a discount of 50% from list on bulbs, tubes or ivory points 30 days – Extra 10% cash in 10 days.
     Can you do better on any reliable brand?
     We enclose stamped envelope and request the favor of a reply. If you can handle our goods we will fill your order immediately. If you are not in a position to do so we will also thank you for the information.
     Trusting we may secure your patronage.
          Very truly yours,
          Richard Slee

The scene is about over, and there is no more

Above: A marketing letter written by Dr. Slee at the turn of the century.

The lab met with official success from the start. A letter from the Pennsylvania State Board of Health brought suggestions and praise for Slee's work. After reviewing plans for the laboratory, George G. Groff, M.D., chairman of the Committee on Preventable Diseases for the board in Lewisburg, Pennsylvania, advised Slee that he would have to extend waste pipes to the operating room and laboratory and should not provide running water behind the animals, as it might make the stables too damp. In a second letter dated 4 days later, Groff wrote that he was "glad to learn you are so fully qualified for the valuable work you have undertaken. Your competition are good business men, but they have not the scientific preparation you possess."

A subsequent inspection by the board of health in July netted Slee more praise. "All operations," the board wrote, "are conducted with the strict attention to asepsis which characterizes modern surgery." The first glycerinated smallpox vaccine was marketed in 1898.

Slee's competition may have been good men, but their products suffered from the same limitations that drove Slee and Sternberg to France in the first place. One problem was infection at the inoculation site. Another was preserving the live virus until it could be given to the patient. Many times, tubes of virus vaccine were found to be inert after they had gotten to market. Slee's glycerinated formula gave his product greater reliability and a longer shelf life.

Dr. E. H. Dickie, of Homer City, Pennsylvania, put the problem in perspective in a letter to Slee in which he asked for samples of the Pocono vaccine. Comparing Slee's product with the competition, Dickie reported failure rates of 30% to 35% using the Parke–Davis vaccine and 10% using product from Mulford Biological Laboratories. Ironically, H. K. Mulford would become the director of research laboratories for the National Drug Co. and would buy Slee's facility 30 years later. As a footnote, Mulford's Laboratories were one of the forerunners of a future partner and competitor, Merck & Co.

Slee included endorsements like Dr. Dickie's in letters he wrote to state boards of health. Although his marketing may have been primitive, his scientific approach to commercializing the business was not. In a letter to the secretary

18

general of the U.S. Navy in Washington, D.C., that March, Slee enclosed samples "of our glycerinated vaccine virus, packed in our latest and what we consider the most scientific form of any on the market." He was referring to the bulb.

Slee had managed three innovations with his vaccine. One was its relative freedom from unpleasant local reactions. The second was an innovation in packaging. He used a Sternberg Bulb, created by his mentor but named by Slee. An editorial in the March 12, 1898, issue of the *Philadelphia Medical Journal* aptly describes the invention: "Only one end is sealed, so that heat cannot destroy the vaccine, as it is very liable to do when both ends are sealed. There is no need of blowing the vaccine through a rubber

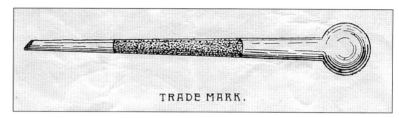

TRADE MARK.

tube with the possibility of infecting it, not by the expired air, but by the sputum, mustache, etc. For using, the point is broken off and the vaccine forced out by the flame of a match applied to the bulb or even by the heat of the hand. It is a happy thought."

The third innovation was an advance in the lab's manufacturing techniques that guaranteed consistency, as Slee noted in a letter that year to Joseph Y. Porter, M.D., state health officer in Jacksonville, Florida: "We especially desire to call your attention to the fact that our virus is mixed by mechanical means which insures every portion of each vial to possess the certainty as to the power of each vial, provided the vaccinator uses care in his work."

The vaccine was not without problems. The state board of health in Philadelphia suggested Slee change the formulation to reduce sore arms on those vaccinated. And the Chicago Board of Health found that the lymph in a Sternberg Bulb "gave an abundant growth of white pus cocci on streak agar, demonstrating that it had not been exposed to the inhibitive action of the glycerin sufficiently long." But for the most part, the new vaccine met with general acceptance, and orders began to arrive in Swiftwater.

In 1898, a year after William McKinley took office as president and songwriters penned "On the Banks of the Wabash," Richard Slee got his first big break. The U.S. battleship *Maine* mysteriously exploded in Havana harbor and America declared war on Spain. By July, Slee was shipping his new vaccine to the troops in Cuba on the hospital ship *Relief*. Although the conflict lasted only 3 months, Slee supplied nearly all of the vaccine used by the U.S. Army. After the war, the needs of occupation forces in Cuba, Puerto Rico, and the Philippines meant a steady demand for his product.

Flush with that success, Slee took steps to broaden distribution, writing in

Above: One of Slee's breakthroughs in manufacturing, the Sternberg Bulb.

August 1898 to Dr. W. Royal Stokes, city bacteriologist with the Health Department in Baltimore, Maryland, for an appointment to discuss his results. They were impressive, if anecdotal. Slee also won the support of the secretary of the Pennsylvania State Board of Health, Dr. Benjamin Lee, who had inoculated his own child with the Pocono vaccine with favorable results.

Business at Swiftwater continued to grow. Slee had made an offer that for $1, he would send a sample of the vaccine to anyone. By the fall, he was receiving inquiries from as far away as Winnipeg, Manitoba. The reports were positive. "We would say," wrote Willet Brown and E. S. Dawson Jr. of Brown & Dawson, druggists and dealers in surgical instruments of Syracuse, New York, "out of the thousands of points that we have used, of yours we have had but very little trouble."

Slee continued to expand his market, although the records show he relied heavily on government purchases from the military and state health services. He wanted to expand further, into production of diphtheria and tetanus antitoxins, but the continued demand for his smallpox vaccine and the funding that such a move would take forced him to put those plans on hold. In early 1899, Lee wrote to Slee that smallpox was widespread in Puerto Rico, but vaccination had never been performed to any extent. Slee sent samples of his vaccine. He also solicited doctors, druggists, local and state boards of health in the United States and Canada, and advertised in medical journals in his attempt to develop more of a demand.

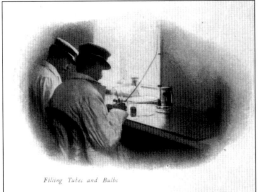

Filling Tubes and Bulbs

THE effect of adding diluted glycerine to the pulp taken from the vaccinated calf is to set up a process of purification in the mixture that advances gradually until a condition is reached where the product may be said to be practically sterile and yet active, so far as vaccination is concerned. This constitutes

The Philadelphia Board of Health placed four orders totaling 5,000 tubes of vaccine during September 1898 and was billed $250. The Manitoba Board of Health in Winnipeg, Canada, began using the vaccine. In a handwritten note on the bottom of a letter from the Indiana Board of Health, Slee said, "The demand for vaccine has been so great that we have had to postpone our antitoxin branch for the present."

By the following year, orders were rolling in, up to 500 tubes per order. Reports were favorable, with many boards of health citing high success rates. Vaccine was sold over a wide area, from Georgia to Iowa, and in several provinces and cities in Canada.

During the latter

Above: Filling tubes and Sternberg Bulbs, from Slee's brochure of 1903.

Right: Orders arrived by telegraph and mail.

THE WESTERN UNION TELEGRAPH COMPANY.

part of December 1899, Lee suggested to the U.S. Commission for the Paris Exposition that Slee's vaccine might be exhibited as a product from Pennsylvania. Slee reproduced a copy of the medals he won in his advertising.

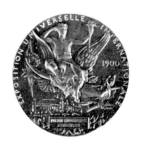

While demand for the product continued to increase, profits did not. The price for 2 dozen doses of the vaccine virus was 25 cents. That included Sternberg Bulbs, capillary tubes, and ivory points. Accurate financial records are not available for 1898, the first full year of operation, but those that exist show sales of $2,060, with expenses of $2,960. This would indicate more than 40,000 doses of vaccine were sold the first year. Expenses ranged from $43.76 for 2,000 stamped envelopes to $7.50 for cigars to $3 for a calf — Slee rented them for the duration of the vaccination process, then returned the animals to the farmer. An account of the early days of the laboratories, published in an Easton newspaper, stated that Slee had five employees. Although there are no authentic records

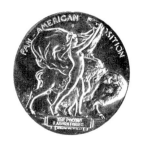

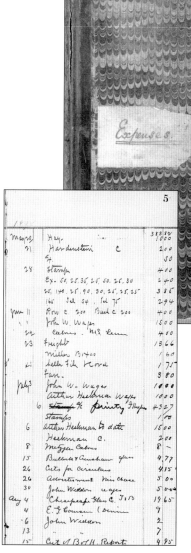

to validate this statement, Slee's journal entries for 1898 show that wages were paid to two men, John Widdoss and Arthur Hartman, and not always on a full-time basis.

With the laboratories in a tight financial position, Slee decided to moonlight. As early as 1897, he began serving as assistant bacteriologist and deputy inspector for the Pennsylvania State Board of Health in the region. As he did with the laboratories, Slee took his public health work seriously. He lobbied state officials to have a coroner appointed in Monroe County, and to have several autopsies performed.

Dr. Lee, the secretary of the State Board of Health, agreed in theory. In a letter dated March 5, 1897, he told Slee, "It is certainly very desirable that that position should be filled by a physician rather than by one of the ignorant class who are so apt to receive such appointments." Two weeks later, Lee advised there was little the two of them could do in the matter. "These cases of failure to hold inquests which you report certainly indicate a very lax condition of county government. At the same time, they are rather legal than sanitary derelictions, and I do not see that our Board can interfere."

By June of that year, Slee was writing to the governor of Pennsylvania concerning the appointment of a coroner, and still getting nowhere. He did make headway on another front: the quarantine of children with measles. In a March 1897 letter to Slee, Lee

Top: Medals Slee won in Paris, 1899.

Left: Slee's ledger of his first three years in business; a page showing expenses from 1898.

laid out a plan of action. "I send you a package of our circulars on measles for distribution. It would be well to get the papers to publish these either in full or

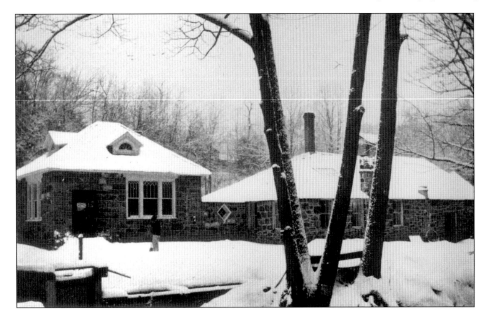

by abstract. I advise your sending each member of the school board a communication accompanying a copy of the circular, urging upon the board the importance of exercising its full authority in forbidding children either just recovered from measles, or members of families in which the disease exists, from attending school."

Slee may not have met with initial success, but that did not stop him from continuing a lifelong quest for new regulations regarding public health.

Partners

As the twentieth century dawned, the country changed from a rural to a more urban place. The automobile gained popularity. Teddy Roosevelt took over as president and ordered construction of the Panama Canal. In Philadelphia, the pharmaceutical industry began to grow with the formation of the National Drug Co. In Swiftwater, the entrepreneurial spirit that had fired Richard Slee had begun to wear thin, tempered by the realities of business. Competition was increasing. Tests showed some of Slee's vaccine was unreliable. The doctor needed to expand, to buy land and equipment, but he needed cash to do so.

He faced the situation by mounting a direct-mail campaign to all parts of the country, extolling the virtues of his vaccine and offering to "deliver all goods free, pay telegraphy and return charges . . . and offer you a discount of 50% from list on bulbs, tubes, or ivory points [if paid for in] 30 days — extra 10% cash [if paid for] in 10 days." He also increased his moonlighting. By 1900, Slee had been promoted to bacteriologist for the Pennsylvania State Board of Health and was earning $15 per day for work and $7.50 for each sample examined "chemically and bacteriologically."

The efforts still were not enough. His contacts, however, were. In 1897, William Redwood Fisher, chief of staff of New York City's Bellevue Hospital,

Above: Pocono Laboratories in winter, circa 1903.

Facing page: Bill from Warner Dry Goods, circa 1900.

decided that because of declining health, he would seek the country air by building a brownstone in Swiftwater, at the juncture of Routes 314 and 611, a site now occupied by Kelly Antiques. Before he retired from private practice in Hoboken, New Jersey, Fisher tried Slee's new vaccine and liked the results, so much so that on January 4, 1901, he wrote to Slee that he had "vaccinated near-ly 200 persons, without a failure in primary cases, and without severe reaction in any case. I consider the vaccine virus of the Pocono Laboratories the surest and the safest in the market."

Less than 3 months later, Slee and Fisher signed a partnership agreement drafted by A. Mitchell Palmer, the Stroudsburg lawyer who would later become attorney general of the United States. Palmer was paid $73.33 for his work. The pair signed the agreement for the purpose of promoting "the art, trade, and business of manufacturing and selling vaccines, anti-toxins, chemicals, and drugs, etc. in the village of Swiftwater."

Fisher was born in 1844 in Mobile, Ala. Four years later, his father, Samuel S. Fisher, died of yellow fever, and the family moved to Philadelphia. Fisher gradu-ated from Columbia College in 1863 and studied at the College of Physicians and Surgeons. He served as chief of staff at Bellevue Hospital, then superinten-dent of the Inebriate Asylum on Ward's Island. He settled in Hoboken in 1874, where he became consulting physician at Christ Hospital in Jersey City, and attending surgeon at St. Mary's Hospital in Hoboken. He was also the medical officer for the Hoboken Ferry Co., North Hudson Co. Railroad, the Morris and Essex Division of the Lackawanna Railroad, the Holland–American Steamship Line, and the Scandinavian–American Steamship Line. In addi-tion, he had a large general practice.

While Fisher had expertise in both medicine and manage-ment, he offered something Slee needed even more — money. Slee had been unable to pay wages on time. Often, he divided the payments. In 1901, John Widdoss earned $30 for a month's work. Slee wrote him a check for $25 in early June and one for $5 at the end of the month.

Fisher got started immediately, pumping capital into the new company. A journal entry for June 1901 shows Fisher wrote a check for $162.44 "to pay expenditures prior to May 1," and a second for $135.00 for the same purpose.

The new relationship allowed Swiftwater's owners to take care of their families. Fisher's two daughters, Elizabeth and Ester, were

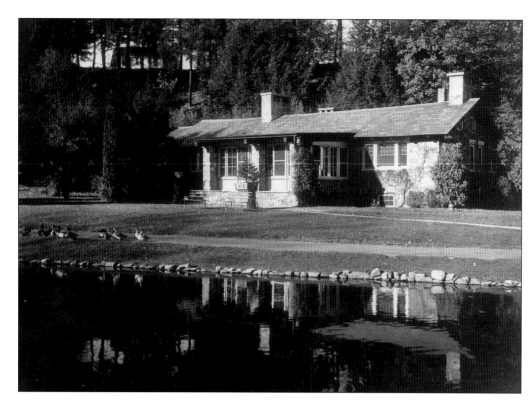

paid $10 each for packing, the first recorded use of female employees on a regular basis. William H. Kent was paid $72.50 for plastering, $27 of which was allocated to the farm and the remaining $45.50 to the Swiftwater Inn. Slee also purchased $108.50 in coal, of which $42.50 was

for the lab and the remaining $66 went to Dr. Fisher.

A listing on December 1901 is the first showing that wages were paid to more than one person. Benjamin Strunk received $25, John H. Widdoss $26 in two payments, and John H. Woodling $39.75 for November and December. Occasional checks of $100 to $500 were made out to Drs. Slee and Fisher, without the reason being stipulated.

A tax notice from the turn of the century lists Slee's holdings as 4 acres of land and buildings, 2 horses and mules, and 1 dog, assessed for Monroe County tax purposes at $1,500, on which Slee paid $3.50 in county tax, $2.10 in school tax, and $1.50 for a dog tax.

Fisher's presence was felt immediately. To compete with the growing number of biological labs, Slee needed to expand. He wanted more land so new calves could be isolated and observed prior to their being vaccinated. In December 1901, Mrs. Annie Bush agreed to sell her 100-acre farm next to the laboratory to Slee and Fisher for $600, a price that was paid by Fisher. He was reimbursed the following year. The farm was transferred in January 1902, with half of the property being listed in the name of each of the co-partners. Slee's section of 50 acres sat at the western end, closest to the laboratory, while Fisher's 49 acres was at the eastern end. For a $15 fee, Palmer prepared the deeds.

Slee also wanted a mechanized way to grind the vaccine lymph that was harvested from the calves. In June 1900, he purchased a waterwheel, 6 feet in diameter, for $88.55. It was powered by water from the dam in the Swiftwater

Above: Bldg. 1, the bachelor quarters, circa 1913.

Facing page:

Top: Deed for land transaction between Mrs. Bush and Dr. Fisher.

Center: Exterior of Slee brochure, 1903.

Bottom: Interior of 1903 brochure.

24

Creek, adjacent to the laboratory.

Over the next 2 years, Slee added an annex, a 23' by 27' office with 18" walls of local stone and a slate roof, and built "Ivy," his home on the hill adjacent to the road, where Building 45 now stands. The interior of the office was finished in polished hardwood, with two desks from the Fred Macy Company Ltd. Slee even formed his own utility, the Swiftwater Water and Power Co., in 1902, with himself as president, his wife Ella as secretary, and Fisher as treasurer.

Fisher's money provided a means of expansion, but it could not limit the rising tide of competition. The federal government had yet to control or license biological laboratories. It was not until 1902 that Congress passed the Biologicals Control Law, and August 1903 that the U.S. Secretary of the

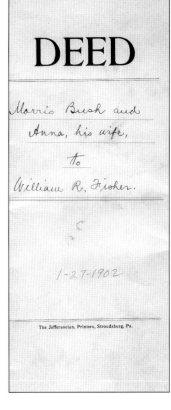

Treasury regulated "the sale of viruses, serums, toxins, and analogous products." Twelve licenses were issued for 1 year to 11 manufacturers, including Parke–Davis & Co., H. K. Mulford Company, and the Pasteur Institute. Pocono Biological Laboratories received license number 6. Of the 11 manufacturers, 7 received licenses to produce

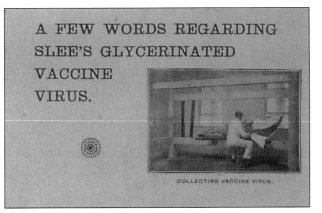

vaccine virus, including the Pocono labs. The competition had begun.

Slee increased the advertising budget, spending $244 in 1903 to print 5,000 illustrated booklets called *A Few Words Regarding Slee's Glycerinated Vaccine Virus.* "The past two years have witnessed a complete revolution in America with regard to the production and marketing of Vaccine Virus," Slee wrote in his introduction. "We feel a pardonable pride in being the first to introduce to the medical profession of this continent the now celebrated 'Glycerinated Pulp Vaccine,' and the accompanying testimonials. . . ."

Queries arrived from across the United States and around the world, including Samoa. Yet despite the interest in the glycerinated product, it was still not enough to support the laboratory, and the partners dissolved their agreement in December 1907. Onlookers might have called it the end of an era. But they would have underestimated the tenacity of Dr. Richard Slee.

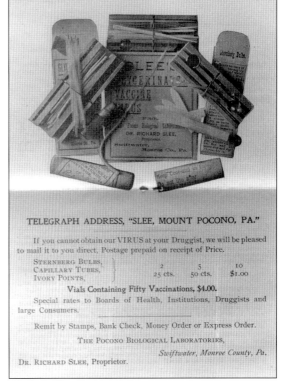

Lederle Calling

With the Knickerbocker Trust Co. and other financial institutions failing in a currency panic that swept the nation in 1907, Slee sought his fortunes elsewhere. In 1908, he closed the Swiftwater facility and moved to New York to direct the production of biological products at the Lederle Antitoxin Laboratory in Pearl River, N.Y. There, Slee had the opportunity to work with the founder of the laboratories, Dr.

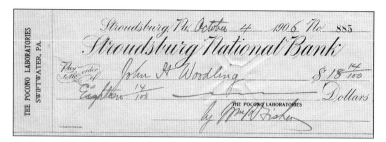

Ernst Lederle, former commissioner of health of New York City, and another researcher who would play a significant role in his future, Dr. Wallace C. Abbott, founder of the forerunner of Abbott Laboratories. The Swiftwater story came to a temporary halt when license number 6, for glycerinated smallpox vaccine, was retired on July 1, 1908.

Even with a tacit endorsement from the federal government, the fledgling biologicals industry still faced a daunting problem not related to finance — a public backlash against vaccination. Despite the reduction in mortality that immunization had brought to the nation, not all of its citizens were convinced this was good public policy, or even effective health care.

In 1908, a medical doctor from Niagara Falls, New York, J. W. Hodge, wrote that compulsory vaccination was "the crime of the century," citing evidence that the process not only violated an American's freedom but that it was ineffective. "The accumulated experience of more than one hundred years has conclusively demonstrated that vaccinia neither prevents smallpox nor mitigates that disease when it attacks the vaccinated."

Slee countered those attacks and others in a letter to the Bergen County, New Jersey, Medical Society in 1910:

Above: John
Woodling's paycheck.

Facing page: Dr.
Richard Slee joins the
nation's first Army
Medical Corps.

> The growth of the anti-vaccination societies in this country is largely due to the undeniable fact that the protection by vaccination was sometimes followed by results that were more serious than would be a mild attack of smallpox. We are now passing through the transition state, so to speak, and in a short time physicians will begin to realize that the regulations of the government are wise and that the failures from time to time are more than offset by the undeniable elimination of many severe and unpleasant sequelae.

As he had done in Swiftwater, Slee felt compelled to go beyond the confines of work. When the U.S. Army created its first reserve unit, the Medical Reserve Corps, Slee became one of the first to be commissioned in the new group. It was as if he could see the forthcoming war in Europe. Then, in 1910, when Dr. Lederle left Pearl River to once again serve as New York City's commissioner of health, Slee struck out on his own for the last time.

Serving the Country (1911–26)

In 1911, Richard Slee returned to Swiftwater without Dr. Fisher and reopened the facility under the name of the Slee Laboratories. He took as his partner his 17-year-old son, Arthur. License number 6 was reissued on July 1, 1912.

During his years at Lederle, Slee had helped to produce an improved version of an impure and expensive diphtheria antitoxin. He also carefully watched the addition of tetanus antitoxin and typhoid vaccine to Lederle's product list. In control of his business once again, Slee expanded production from a sole product, smallpox vaccine. In 1912, he was licensed to produce human tetanus antitoxin. To do that, he needed horses, which would be bled for serum. That liquid would be refined for its antibodies, then used to transfer immunity to humans. He remodeled the former calf barn to stable 8 horses, constructed a new smallpox calf unit (Building 2), and expanded the staff.

In the years leading up to World War I, Slee produced diphtheria antitoxin; veterinary tetanus antitoxin; antimeningitis serum; antistreptococcic serum; normal serum; vaccine serum; anticanine distemper vaccine; antityphoid vaccine typhus and paratyphoid; and antityphoid vaccine typhoid.

Even with a broader product line, Slee still faced the old problem of finding sales and distribution channels. Using his contacts at Lederle, he formed an agreement with Wallace Abbott, then president of the Abbott Alkaloidal Co. in Chicago, to market the products of the Swiftwater Labs.

With the arrangement came increased work. Aside from the death of his father in 1912, the times were good to Richard. He listed nine people on the payroll the following year and began assuming more duties, including that of sanitary officer, with the Army Reserve Medical Corps. With increased distribution, more horses were required, and in 1913–14 Slee built a new stone stable for 20 horses, complete with operating room (Building 6A). The Slees began producing gas gangrene antitoxin and developed a sideline of K prophylactic packets, primarily for the armed forces.

At the same time, Richard and Ella built a house to replace Ivy, the Slee's

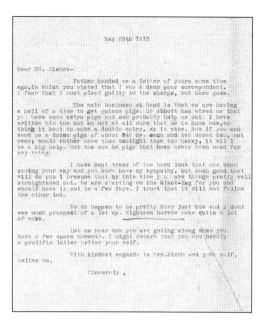

May 29th 1915

Dear DR. Biehn:-

Father handed me a letter of yours some time ago, in which you stated that I was a damn poor corospondent. I fear that I must plead guilty to the charge, but hare goes.

The main business at hand is that we are having a hell of a time to get guinea pigs. Dr Abbott has wired us that yo have some extra pigs and can probably help us out. I have written him too but am not at all sure that he is home now, so think it best to make a double entry, as it were. Now if you can send us a dozen pigs of about 340 Gr. each and two dosen 240, not over; would rather have them toolight than too heavy, it wil l be a big help. but the mus be pigs that have never been used for any thing.

I have kept track of the hard luck that has been coming your way and you sure have my sympathy, but much good that will do you I presume that by this time you have things pretty well streightened out. We are starting on the Black-leg for you and should have it out in a few days. I trust that it will not follow the other lot.

We do happen to be pretty busy just now and I dont see much prospect of a let up. Eighteen horses make quite a lot of work.

Let me hear how you are getting along when you have a few spare moments. I might remark that you are hardly a prolific latter writer your self.

With kindest regards to Mrs.Biehn and your self, Belive me,

Sincerely ,

Above: Arthur Slee's letter to Dr. J. F. Biehm.

Facing page: 1st Lt. Richard Slee, left, and 1st Lt. C. I. Wertenbaker of the U.S. Army Medical Reserve Corps in camp May 21, 1910, with the 29th U.S. Infantry in East Haven, Conn.

original home, which burned prior to that. That house, called the bungalow or bachelor quarters or Building 1, later housed Human Resources personnel.

The war in Europe began in 1914, but because of the U.S. policy of isolationism, the conflict did not affect the rank and file in America. Life went on for the Slees, too. In 1915, Arthur married Phoebe Edmunds of Lynchburg, Virginia. She was 21 years old and considered by the social set in Monroe County to be the quintessential Southern belle.

Arthur began taking on more responsibility. In a letter to Dr. J. F. Biehm, director of the Abbott Laboratories in Ravenswood, Chicago, Arthur struggled as much with a manual typewriter as he did with the mantle of command. For people who believe that standards of English and composition are continually declining, Arthur's letter of May 29, 1915, reproduced here as he typed it, offers a refreshing view:

Dear DR. Biehn:-

Father handed me a letter of yours some time ago, in which you stated that I was a damn poor corospondent. I fear that I must plead guilty to the charge, but hare goes.

The main business at hand is that we are having a hell of a time to get guinea pigs. Dr Abbott has wired us that you have some extra pigs and can probably help us out. I have written him too but am not at all sure that he is home now, so think it best to make a double entry, as it were. Now if you can send us a dozen pigs of about 340 Gr. each and two dosen 240, not over; would rather have them toolight than too heavy, it wil l be a big help. But the mus be pigs that have never been used for any thing.

We do happen to be pretty busy just now and I dont see much prospect of a let up. Eighteen horses make quite a lot of work.

With kindest regards to Mrs.Biehn and your self,

Belive me,

Sincerely,

Arthur may be excused the sloppy correspondence because he had a lot on his mind. The war in Europe had overwhelmed the laboratories with orders for tetanus antitoxin, diphtheria antitoxin, and smallpox vaccine, so much so that it turned away $800,000 in business that year. New opportunities arose every month. In the spring of 1915, the labs negotiated an agreement with McKesson and Robbins, a New York City firm, to sell biologic products in "Australasia, Philippine Islands, Japan, China, India, Russia, Asia, Africa, and Straits Settlements for the period of five years." The schedule attached to that agreement showed that the Slees were selling 1,000-unit syringes of diphtheria antitoxin for $1.25 each; 1,500 units of human tetanus antitoxin for $2.50 each; 750 units of veterinary tetanus antitoxin for $0.75 each; and 5 tubes of vaccine virus for $0.75.

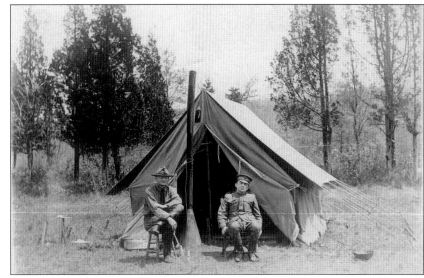

Despite the remoteness of the war for most Americans, its shadow loomed over Swiftwater. As an officer in the Medical Reserve Corps, Richard Slee had written to the War Department to determine if he would see active military service. In a letter dated June 21, 1915, to Dr. Slee, Maj. Robert E. Noble, with the Army Medical Corps, Surgeon General's Office, wrote that, "In case it is necessary to order officers of the Medical Reserve Corps into active duty, I do not think there will be any delay in your receiving an order for active service. You can understand, of course, that your greatest value, at first, would be in aiding the government to obtain a sufficient quantity of the supplies of your laboratories to meet the emergency."

The demands of the war also exhausted Slee's supply of tetanus antitoxin, limited his distribution, and tried his patience. He wrote to Dr. Biehm in October that shipments from Germany of many components crucial to his operation had ceased:

> The war has upset us dreadful in regard to filter paper, Berkfeld filters and other most necessary parts of our trade, so to speak. We are gradually substituting things of our own invention and are getting around the many difficulties. America may be a very bright nation, but between you and I, we are really nothing but a nation of assemblers and we have built up our reputation most largely on adopting European ideas, buying their stock, stamping it together and putting a nickel plate or a polish on it and calling it a product of America. This is rather strong, but it is true.

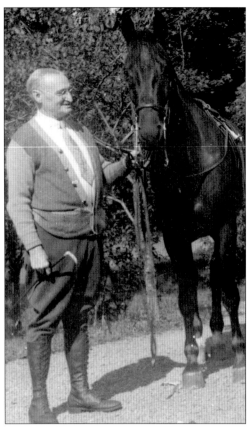

While he could do nothing about the bottleneck in supplies, Slee got his wish for active duty in 1916, when he was ordered to report to Camp Summerall at Tobyhanna, Pennsylvania. He had been eager to serve the military, but what he found resembled George Washington's beleaguered camp at Valley Forge more than the army of a modern nation.

"I found the Camp in wretched condition," he wrote to Maj. Noble on July 31, "everything out of repair, and suffering from the winter storms." As sanitary officer, he was distressed at the lack of training and transportation. But he praised the soldiers for their eagerness to help. "I cannot speak too highly of the treatment which I received at their hands." He did not appreciate their apparent lack of respect for the American flag, and wrote to Col. Robert M. Danford at Camp Summerall on August 28, 1916, after a ceremony of the colors at Tobyhanna: "I was simply disgusted to see any number of civilians 'slouching around' and without any thought of removing their hats during this impressive ceremony."

Slee was commissioned a first lieutenant. He made at least one trip to Washington to lobby on behalf of the new army reorganization bill, even though its passage would abolish the Medical Reserve Corps. He also helped to form an association of vaccine producers who met in New York concerning the setting of uniform board of health prices for biological products, a move that was vetoed strongly by Frank Ryan, the president of Parke–Davis. Slee also kept a running correspondence with Abbott in Chicago and apparently sent him a black horse hide, which Abbott tanned and turned into an automobile robe. Despite their friendship, the business slumped again. Slee confided to Abbott that his effort to cut prices below those of his competitors had resulted in "a decided falling off in sales."

Slee was also concerned about the war and its effect on his business. After encountering trouble when buying glass for syringe barrels, he complained to Abbott in June that, "No one in Washington, from the highest to the lowest, seems to have the faintest idea as to the outcome of the war." He was also having some physical pain, suffering from an old neck wound.

Then more trouble. In late 1916, after several distributors had returned lots of vaccine that were past their expiration date, Slee introduced a new method of sterilization, brilliant green dye, about which few records remain. By year's end, nature turned against him. "We had a very serious cloud burst several weeks ago which destroyed our power plant and washed out our dam," he wrote to

Above: Dr. Richard Slee enjoying his favorite pasttime, in this undated photo.

Facing page, top: Phoebe Slee holds her new son, Richard E.

Facing page, bottom: Swiftwater's office in the late 1920s.

Abbott. In a letter to Dr. Alfred S. Burdick at the Abbott Laboratories, Slee said the situation was creating "a very serious financial loss to us." Burdick was sympathetic. "I am mighty sorry to learn of the injury to your dam."

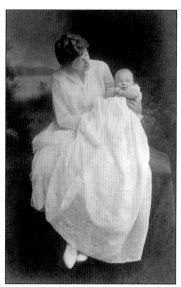

The winter of 1916–17 was not a good one for the Slee family. Arthur became ill, then Ella. Richard suffered with the flu in late 1916, and then in February he wrote to Abbott, "I have not been well for several weeks, with indigestion that has been aggravated by being rather nervous over various things in connection with the work, and the result was that I gave out; had to go to bed on Sunday." He complained about the "continuous severe cold weather" in the Poconos.

By June 1917 he was feeling better. There was promising news in the family, too. His grandson, Richard Edmunds Slee, had been born in March. And, as Richard wrote to Abbott, there was good news on the financial front: Richard Slee expected to receive a raise from $2,000 to $3,000 per year upon his anticipated commission as a major in the Medical Officers Reserve Corps. He accepted the commission on June 9. Meanwhile, Slee was posted to the U.S. Ambulance Corps Camp in Allentown, Pennsylvania. As the United States entered the war and the camp prepared to send ambulances to Europe, Arthur began handling the correspondence from Swiftwater, sharing with Abbott in an August letter his concern over how the war would affect the market. "If we get a large Army in France there is sure to be a great demand for tetanus antitoxin."

Richard remained at his post throughout the war. He was promoted to major at the time he reported for duty, lieutenant-colonel in 1918, and colonel in 1919. When the first commanding officer of Camp Crane left for Italy, Slee succeeded him. He helped to close the camp on April 12.

If the war had been difficult for the Slees, peacetime presented new challenges. Upon their return to civilian life in the 1920s, Richard and Arthur were faced with no means of distributing their products, except through contracts to major purchasers, such as the army and state boards of health. Both the War Department and the navy ordered smallpox vaccine. The Army Supply Base in Brooklyn, New York, became a large purchaser of Slee's vaccines. In January alone, the base ordered 13,420 units of smallpox vac-

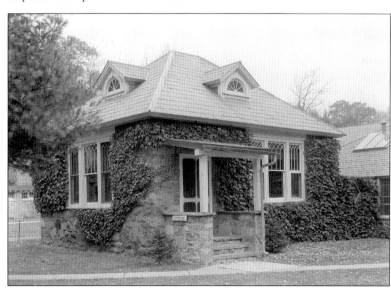

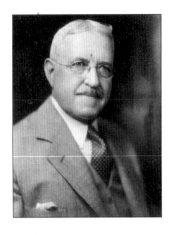

cine, plus vials of diphtheria antitoxin and veterinary tetanus antitoxin. One order, placed by the Naval Medical Supply Depot in Brooklyn, amounted to $927.40.

Dr. Slee continued his active work in the army reserve corps, organizing the General Medical Laboratory No. 1, Slee Laboratory Unit, in 1922. But even his much-anticipated military pay could not offset the lack of work at the labs.

The passing of the torch started in 1926, when H. K. Mulford — a pioneer in the field of biological production and founder of the Mulford Biological Laboratories — accepted the directorship of the Research and Biological Laboratories of the National Drug Co. in Philadelphia. The small laboratory, located on Germantown Avenue, soon proved inadequate. Knowing of Slee's Laboratory in Swiftwater, Mulford negotiated an arrangement whereby National would rent the facilities in 1927 with an option to buy.

Richard Slee had already joined the staff of the New York State Department of Health in 1923, then served as deputy commissioner of health in West Chester County, New York. He remained in White Plains until his retirement in 1937. As for Dr. William Fisher, the former partner in the Pocono Biological Laboratories died at his home in Swiftwater in 1926. He did not live to see the next era at Swiftwater.

Above: H.K. Mulford.

Below: National Drug's sign at the entrance to the Swiftwater Laboratories, in the late 1920s.

The National Years (1927–55)

The American expansion continued. In 1927, Charles A. Lindbergh flew *The Spirit of St. Louis* nonstop across the Atlantic Ocean. The monument at Mount Rushmore was dedicated. The first successful demonstration of television took place in New York City.

National Drug was looking to expand beyond the pharmaceutical business into biologicals and vaccines. It had outgrown its Germantown Avenue laboratory and could not stable large animals like horses and sheep. The lease of the Swiftwater facilities proved to be a good match on both sides, creating a family-like atmosphere that would live on in the memories of its employees even to this day.

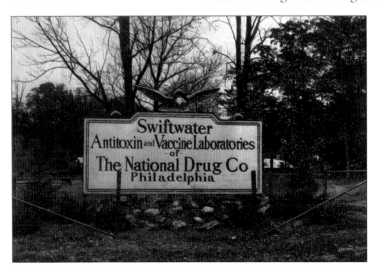

Like Swiftwater, National had a reputation for excellence and for hiring good help. Founded in 1899 by G. F. Harvey of Troy,

New York, and joined a year later by Charles Carr, National began manufacturing pharmaceuticals in 1900 in Philadelphia, with headquarters at 4663 Stenton Avenue. In 1887, H. K. Mulford established a company that developed the first commercially practical diphtheria antitoxin. In 1926, when National decided to expand into biologicals, it hired Mulford as its director of research and laboratories. The next year, Mulford leased the Swiftwater Labs with an

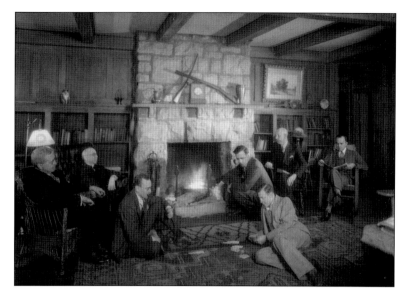

option to buy and hired Russell P. Knerr as director of those biological laboratories. Arthur Slee remained in charge of production. Twelve people worked at Swiftwater at the time.

Eager to expand, National built an isolation unit (Building 8) for the production of tetanus toxin, which the Slees had purchased from Gilliland Laboratory

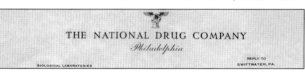

and the New York City Board of Health Laboratory. Additional facilities for 60 horses (Building 6B) were added. So were additional personnel.

National Drug made its ownership official in 1930. On May 26, Richard Slee, his wife, and mother-in-law deeded 46.81 acres of the old Pocono Biological Laboratories to National Drug. Arthur Slee was retained as director of the establishment, serving in that capacity until 1937, when he assumed additional duties as associate director of the Biological Division of National Drug.

The Great Depression

The stock market crash of 1929 and the Great Depression of the early 1930s had little documented effect on National. The 1931 catalogue lists 31 biological products. Facilities for 40 more horses (Building 6C) were added. In the booklet *Five Years of Progress*, written in 1932 by Mulford himself, the director talked of nothing but expansion to the north:

> The Swiftwater Laboratories have shown a remarkable growth and
> development. In 1926 the capacity was limited to the immunization
> of 12 horses — we now carry 72 horses, some in full production;
> others in expansion of high immunization for the preparation

Above: The bachelor quarters at Swiftwater, with, from left, H. K. Mulford, C. P. Brown, Arthur Slee, Warren Rawlings, Russell Knerr, D. H. Bergey, and Clarence Rinker.

Left: National Drug letterhead from the 1930s.

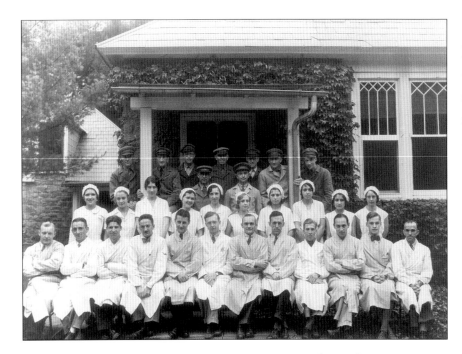

of diphtheria, tetanus and perfringens (gas gangrene) antitoxins, scarlet fever streptococcus antitoxin, refined and extra concentrated pneumonia serum, anti-erysipelas, anti-meningococcic, antistreptococcic and normal serums. Rabies and smallpox vaccines, diphtheria toxoid and toxin-antitoxin mixture are also produced at Swiftwater. Work on antianterior poliomyelitis serum is in progress.

New buildings have been erected, changes and improvement made to former buildings and special equipment provided, laboratories enlarged and personnel strengthened. From the year 1926 to 1931, the staff has continued to grow. Furthermore, members with post-graduate degrees increased by 70%.

Production during the period skyrocketed. From 1930 to 1931, the number of completed packages of biologicals more than doubled, from approximately 68,000 to more than 141,000. Chloroform-killed rabies vaccine and erysipelas serum, used for the acute disease of skin and subcutaneous tissue caused by a species of hemolytic streptococcus, were added to the line. The labs increased the potency of tetanus antitoxin and reduced its loss during the process of concentration.

For the people at Swiftwater, the chores were never done. A policy adopted in 1933 set the workday for "stable men and all other men in exterior work on hourly payroll" at 7 A.M. to 5 P.M., with a half hour for lunch. By state law, women were allowed to work up to 8 hours a day.

By 1934, National had imposed accounting standards on a division that, 30 years earlier, had written undocumented checks to its officers. For the first time, employees had to keep a record of supplies drawn from the stockroom. Transfers from one department to another were recorded. Standards of hygiene and appearance were set, as illustrated in a memo from Arthur Slee in 1935: "Men from the stable visiting the Carr building [Building 4] and other laboratory

Above: Staff photo at the Swiftwater Labs, circa 1932. Arthur Slee is sixth from the right.

Facing page: From left, Elmer Mader, Charley 'Poppy' Mader, Jake Mader, and Dave Coffman tend to the horses outside the main stable, circa 1932. Horses were bled to produce tetanus antitoxin serum.

buildings are to see that loose manure is removed from their shoes and loose hay, straw, and chaff shaken from their clothes before entering these buildings." By 1938, uniforms were required.

While the home-grown look was disappearing from the front office, it flourished in the research department. In an April 1939 article in the *American Journal of Public Health*, D. H. Bergey, Claude P. Brown, and S. Etris published results of toxoid studies on a number of people. Those test subjects were undoubtedly employees of the Swiftwater Labs. In a 1936 letter to David H. Bergey, director of research in biology for National, Arthur Slee wrote that individuals injected in 1934 and 1935 included M. Shick, R. Coffman, Dr. Love, R. Bach, K. Williams, H. Martin, and V. Coffman. Russell Bach was listed as an employee in August 1933. Kenneth Williams was listed as working in culture media production in November 1934. Vincent Coffman worked in the production of rabies and smallpox vaccine during that time. Richard Coffman was one of two night watchmen in January 1935.

Road to Recovery

The latter part of the 1930s reflected the general business slump of the country, as the recovery of 1934 gave way to an economic downturn in 1938. In 1 year, the operating losses at Swiftwater amounted to nearly $50,000. A quiet and frugal man, Arthur Slee became the right person to lead the labs to prosperity. With his campaign hat and riding boots, Slee appeared to outsiders as the flamboyant manager of that mysterious place on the hill, where horses grazed for no apparent reason. To the more familiar eye, Arthur was a retiring man who liked to let his wife host the parties and dispense information on the social graces. He was

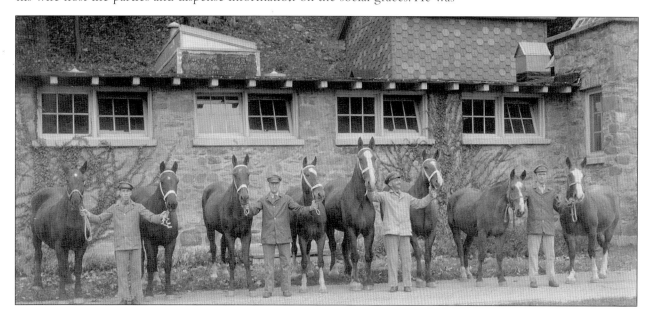

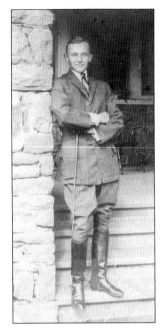

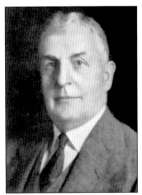

also a shrewd recycler of all things broken and used, a scavenger of the local junkyard for parts that would keep his operation going.

He would regularly drive the 10 miles south to Stroudsburg and visit the bank, the drug store, and occasionally the lounge at the Penn Stroud Hotel on Main Street. While in town, he would usually drop by D. Katz & Sons Inc. and trade with owner David Katz. Slee would scour the yard for small motors, bent iron, and pieces of stainless steel pipe, paying a dollar or two each visit. He would use the material to make supports for his cages or to repair laboratory equipment. For his part, Katz would send a truck to the labs to gather scrap iron, piping, and the broken parts of small-animal cages.

With war looming in Europe again, National Drug began hiring. For Clair Wallingford, fresh out of high school, his first job interview produced both excitement and anxiety. When he arrived at the Swiftwater Labs in February 1938, he found an entrance road lined on both sides with hydrangeas. Building 1 had become a dormitory for single men. There was a pond in front of it, with ducks. The Swiftwater Creek was dammed and formed a waterfall, with a foot-bridge crossing the dam to a pasture where Building 45, the administrative building, now stands. There was a waterwheel in the basement of Building 4, known at the time as the Carr Building, named for former National Drug board chairman Charles E. Carr, the founder of the Twenty Year Club, organized to honor employees with at least 20 years of service. The wheel was used to grind smallpox pulp.

Wallingford's nervousness soon turned into curiosity, then amazement, as he entered the office of Arthur Slee. As Wallingford recalled the office:

Top: Arthur Slee poses with his ever-present riding boots.

Above: Charles Carr.

Right: Offices of the Swiftwater Labs in 1932.

It was paneled in chestnut. The room had a high-beamed ceiling and a stone fireplace. The walls were adorned with guns, swords, pictures, and other memorabilia from World War I. The office was a very dark, dingy place — you might call it —

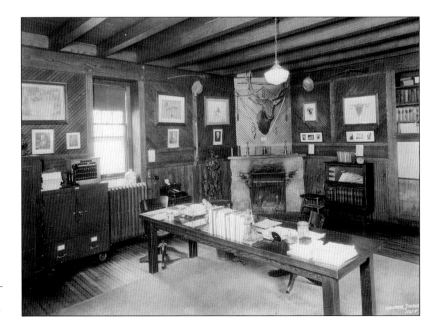

yet Arthur Slee was there, and Merlin Rutt, his secretary. This place
fascinated me because he had all kinds of war things on the wall,
including swords and guns — Arthur's collection from World War I.
To me, it was a beautiful place.

Slee quickly put the young man at ease as he described the work. Wallingford
soon found himself washing bottles and tubes in the kitchen — the area that
prepared media and sterilized equipment for production — for 27 cents an
hour, or $11.88 for a 44-hour week. Through no fault of his own, with the war
and the draft approaching, it was a job he could not keep.

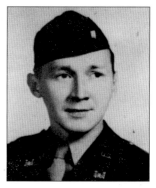

The Science of Patriots (1939–45)

In September 1939, Germany invaded Poland and plunged the world into
another global conflict. While the United States would not enter the war until
the Japanese bombing of Pearl Harbor in 1941, Americans were working to
supply the Allies with materiel and medical supplies. In Swiftwater, the effort
went far beyond that.

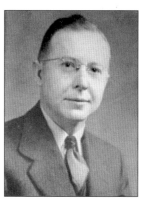

In 1938, fresh from a master's degree program at Lehigh University, Anthony
Bolyn landed at Swiftwater for a brief time, then returned in 1943 with a Ph.D.
from Purdue University and a desire to work in serum processing and with the
diphtheria and gas gangrene group. He worked closely with the "responsible
head" of the establishment, Russell Knerr, to combine diphtheria or tetanus
toxin with antitoxin, then purify the results.

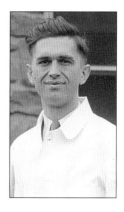

Bolyn and the other single men at Swiftwater lived in Building 1, the Russell
Knerr building, also called
the bungalow. They were
supervised by a house-
mother and cook, who,
when she wasn't looking
after her boys, prepared
duck eggs that she gathered
from the flock by the pond.
The arrangement generated
fond memories and great
science. In April 1944,
Bolyn and his team pro-
duced another break-

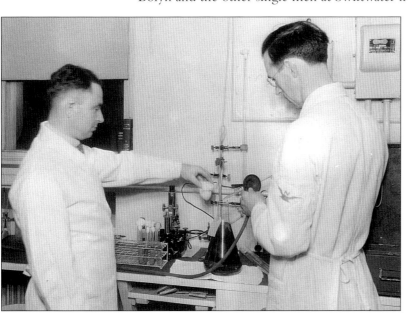

**From top: Clair
Wallingford in
1943; Russell
Knerr; Tony Bolyn
in 1947.**

**Left: Preparing
tetanus antitoxins
at Swiftwater.**

through — the first commercially successful triple-immunization vaccine, DTP, or diphtheria–tetanus–pertussis.

One of the unique characteristics of this combination vaccine was the low incidence of side effects. Similar vaccines of the time contained alum, which was used as a precipitant for the toxoid. The original preparation contained half a percent of alum. When the injection was given, many people developed a large nodule or an ulcer. Bolyn discovered he could greatly reduce the amount of alum, thereby decreasing the side effects.

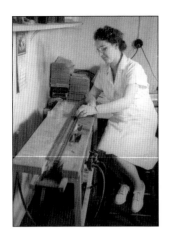

The bombing of Pearl Harbor in 1941 brought new business and a mild sense of paranoia to the labs. As America entered the war, the demand for biological products ballooned and laboratory facilities were tripled. The horse population swelled to better than 500, most of which were housed in the Long Pond area. Production increased fivefold. Additions were constructed on Buildings 2 and 3. New structures went up — Buildings 11 and 12, plus stables 6D and 6E.

The fear and excitement of global conflict eventually found its way to the laboratories in Swiftwater. On December 12, 1941, a memo to workers cautioned them not to "become hysterical over this situation" but to be prepared for "the unexpected. . . . Remember Pearl Harbor." It went on to say that each employee would be furnished with an identification card and that, "It is the duty of every employee to challenge every and any individual found on the premises and demand his or her credentials, if they are not in evidence."

Above: Margaret Butz operates a device that automatically seals capillary tubes in this photo taken in the 1940s.

Below: Merlin Rutt and Ellen Regan in the executive offices, December 1944.

Life at Swiftwater became hectic. There were shortages of people and materials. The labs had been supplying not only the Red Cross but the French and British governments. After 1941, almost the entire output of the laboratories went to U.S. armed forces. Despite Arthur Slee's intervention with the local draft board, Clair Wallingford was commissioned as a second lieutenant and stationed in the South Pacific. His father, James, who worked in maintenance at the time, wrote to his son that the plant could not produce vaccine quickly enough.

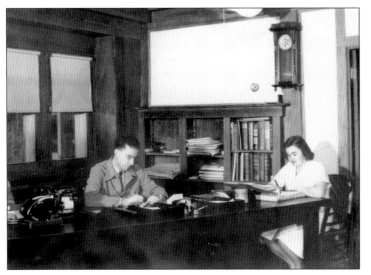

Clair recalled the extraordinary effort made by the people in Swiftwater at the time. "For the smallpox vaccine, they used a needle that went into glass tubing. They used to send them home. My mom and dad worked nights to stick the needles in this glass tubing. They'd

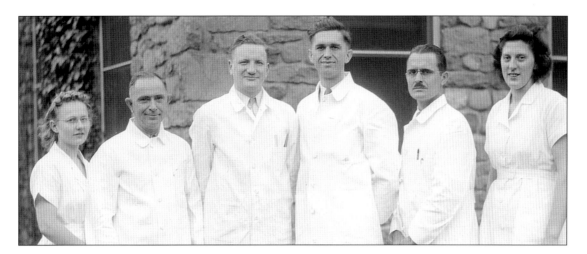

take them back to the lab the next day to be sealed and sterilized. All the employees took them home. I think we got a quarter for a bundle. At least we were helping the war effort."

"The place was going like crazy," said Ellen Regan, who joined Swiftwater straight out of high school in 1942. "There was a smallpox scare. Smallpox vaccine was put up in capillary tubes, one drop in each tube. We filled smallpox vaccine in vials — small ones — because they needed it that fast. Everyone worked together in the production building. Everybody worked 7 days a week. The company brought in your dinner for you. [The workers] were happy that they had done something for their country. That's the way they were."

Regan joined the labs as a finisher, then worked as a secretary for Knerr. She maintained immunization and bleeding records for up to 500 horses. But her fame spread when she took over operation of the company switchboard, poking her head out the window to greet visitors as they drove onto the property.

Despite the urgency of the times, the employees humanized their workplace. There were picnics, blood drives, and war bond rallies, plus regular updates in the *National Bulletin,* the company's employee publication, concerning the exploits of the Swiftwater bowling team.

By Christmas 1942, the workers in Swiftwater had decided they'd already paid the price of war. In a letter to the editor of the *National Bulletin*, a person known only as "Lonesome" showed that Arthur Slee was not the only employee concerned with the effects of the draft.

Above: The staff of the Swiftwater Labs in 1947: From left, Lorraine Rustine, Russell Bach, Martin Yanishevsky, Anthony Bolyn, Russell Stout, and Helen Butz.

Below: In the early 1940s, workers sealed capillary tubes of smallpox vaccine by hand.

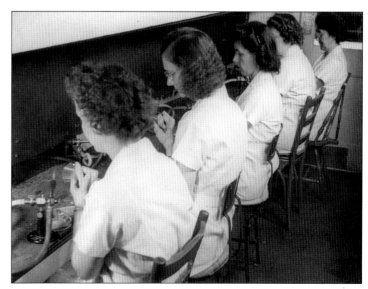

The Swiftwater girls have been good all year, and are now putting in their Christmas requests. We have decided that the single male stock has depleted and would like to put in a requisition for new eligible material.

The qualifications are between the ages of 20 and 26, high, wide, handsome, single, and hitting on all six cylinders. If any of the applicants are deficient in any vitamins, come along as the Swiftwater National Drug will remedy the condition. You see, we are thinking of the Company, too.

"Lonesome"

(Ed. note: If Lonesome can supply a set of genuine pre-war silk stockings, sheer, size 20, for hanging over her Xmas fireplace, editor will guarantee 1 single 6-cylinder male for a Christmas present.)

Below: Cover of National's employee publication from 1945, showing the presentation of the coveted Army–Navy 'E' award to the Swiftwater Labs.

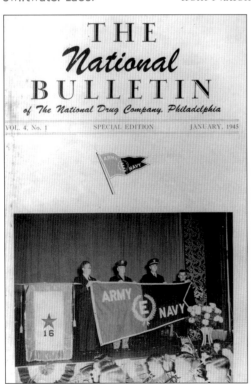

THE *National* BULLETIN
of The National Drug Company, Philadelphia

VOL. 4, No. 1   SPECIAL EDITION   JANUARY, 1945

Finally, in 1944, the hard work paid off. The Swiftwater Laboratories received the coveted Army–Navy "E" award. They became one of a select group, representing less than 2% of the suppliers to the armed forces, to receive that award. In making the presentation, Lt. Col. R. R. Patch of the U.S. Surgeon General's office said the mass tetanus toxoid immunization program of U.S. armed forces in the summer of 1941 had shown no reactions in men immunized with toxoid from National Drug. The toxoid of other manufacturers produced reactions.

A study was instituted that enabled other manufacturers to produce products comparable to National's, due in large part to Tony Bolyn, who shared the trade secret for the war effort. At the time, Swiftwater was producing enough toxoid to immunize nearly 50% of America's armed forces. At ceremonies on December 6, James Wallingford, father of Clair, represented the employees in accepting the "E" flag.

The conclusion of the war signaled a series of endings and beginnings for Swiftwater and the Slee family. Arthur relinquished active supervision of the production laboratories and established headquarters at the main office in Philadelphia as director of the Biological Division. He devoted much of his time to liaison work with officials in Washington, D.C. His son, Richard E. Slee, married Mary Waldron Sisco in 1941. The news turned sad in 1943, with the death of Arthur's mother, Ella. Then, on April 8, 1945, Dr. Richard M. Slee, the founder of the

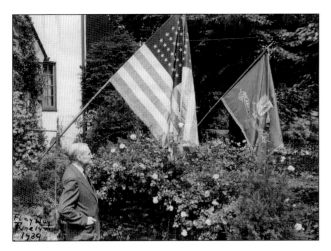

Swiftwater Labs, died. A former deputy commissioner of health in West Chester County, New York, he had retired in 1937 and returned to Monroe County to live out his remaining years. All was not bitter that summer. Three months later, in July, Deborah Waldron Slee, daughter of Richard E. and Mary Slee, was born in Harrisburg. As the war ended overseas, the Slee family entered its fourth generation in America.

The Postwar Years

Most of the government contracts ended shortly after the war, and the laboratory was left with a huge inventory of antitoxins. In addition to the inventory, medical science had moved forward with the development of chemotherapeutic agents, such as the sulfonamides, and the antibiotic penicillin. Many felt the demand for vaccines and antitoxins would drop. Arthur Slee retired in 1945 and returned to Monroe County; Russell Knerr was appointed director of biologicals. National considered major cutbacks, even closing the Swiftwater facility.

A review of sales figures convinced them otherwise.

"Now that peace has been declared and most of the war contracts have been terminated, no doubt you are concerned about the prospects of your company and your own future," the *National Bulletin* reported in September 1945. "We have experienced our largest growth since 1940, and during the past 5 years we have doubled our normal business."

By 1947, income from National's biological operations exceeded the company's pharmaceutical sales. National added to Building 3. It started production of immune globulin from placentas in Building 6A–B and influenza virus vaccine in chicken embryos in Building 6B. The latter was a government contract for which no license was issued. Labeling operations were transferred from Swiftwater to Philadelphia.

Logic and the experience of the Slees after World War I should have lead National

Above: Dr. Richard Slee on Flag Day, June 14, 1939.

Below: From left, Walt Strunk, Clair Wallingford, and Clifford Okuno provide a demonstration at the armory in East Stroudsburg, Pennsylvania, circa 1947.

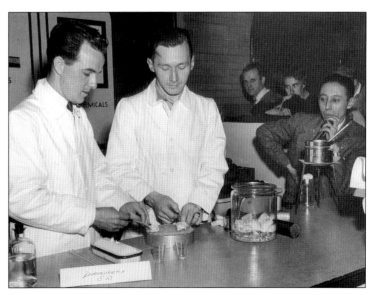

into a retrenchment program. But as GIs flooded home and started the baby boom, America's view of health care began to change, as noted in a National study a few years later:

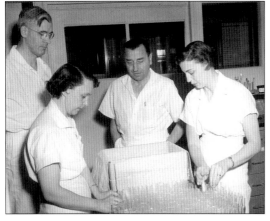

Two pictures document the visit to Swiftwater of yellow fever expert Dr. Gelain Courtrois of the Belgian Congo. Top, from left: Willard Webster, Edith Wilson, Courtrois, and Gerry Parr. Bottom, from left: Anthony Bolyn, assistant director of the labs; Leland Baker, associate director; Courtrois; Webster, in charge of YF vaccine production; and Clifford Okuno, director of Quality Control.

Pediatric immunization is a field showing increasing growth. Parents now request that their children be immunized in contrast to their past reluctance. In addition, there has been an unexpected rise in the birth rate for the past 5 years, which has contributed in part to an increase of 10 million in the population of the country.

The American public is becoming better informed through current periodicals, movies, and broadcasts about the "shots" that they formerly dreaded and now more than often request.

The war was the greatest test of the efficacy of biologics.

A closer solution to the problems connected with immunization against the common cold, infantile paralysis, and tuberculosis challenges our imagination regarding future markets when the final answers are obtained.

Finally, *prevention* will ever be more desired than *cure*. The future of immunizing products still appears long and bright.

The Man Who Built Swiftwater

When G. Willard Webster arrived in 1950, Swiftwater had just obtained a contract to produce Japanese B encephalitis vaccine in chicken embryos for the U.S. government. It was supposed to be a freeze-dried product, and that required new technology for the labs. The original freeze-dryers were open and constantly springing leaks.

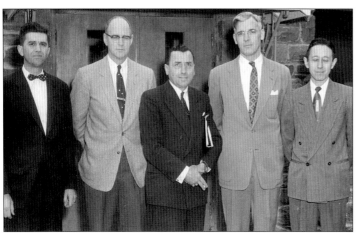

"The first encephalitis vaccine gave us trouble because we didn't have any equipment that worked," Webster recalled. "We got into a government contract and they wanted a freeze-dryer. We were trying to freeze-dry materials without much success."

Webster, who pioneered the process in 1938 at Sharp & Dohme and refined it later at the University of Pennsylvania, introduced a closed-chamber system. It worked. There were

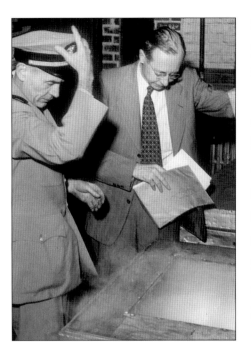

four freeze-dryers from a firm in Philadelphia that did not perform adequately. He developed a new system and began taking on new work.

Over the decades, Webster, who rose to become assistant director of manufacturing for National Drug, brought yellow fever and epidemic typhus vaccine production to the company. He helped to secure a license for epidemic typhus vaccine, issued in 1951. In 1952, his actions allowed Swiftwater Laboratories to become the sole American manufacturer of yellow fever vaccine, assuming the work from the U.S. Public Health Service. He helped to build a new isolation unit; a product license was issued in 1953. He mechanized the filling and labeling department.

Webster also worked with Dr. Jonas Salk and put together crash programs to meet several flu epidemics. But his lasting impact on the company can be seen throughout the campus in its buildings: He helped design and construct virtually all of Swiftwater's manufacturing facilities.

"He was the guiding light and oversaw the planning, construction, and remodeling of most buildings on campus," said Dr. Don Metzgar, who joined National Drug in 1966 as senior virologist and retired in 1994 as senior vice president of Connaught Laboratories Ltd., Swiftwater's parent company from 1978 to 1989. "Willard had a hand in designing and running almost all of the buildings back to the yellow fever building. His involvement could earn him the title of 'The Man Who Built Swiftwater.'"

Before he retired in 1978, Webster had planned the construction of Building 14 (yellow fever), Building 21 (the pertussis laboratory), Building 32 (named the Bolyn Building for Quality Control), Building 37 (dedicated as the Webster building for influenza vaccine production), and Building 38 (the addition to Building 37 for warehouse and distribution).

Webster enjoyed the work. "It was very satisfying. I got a great kick out of laying them out. A couple of times I came out pretty well on the cost, although I never pretended to be an architect."

Left: Lt. Cmdr. Murphy, left, and Russell Knerr inspect a shipment of yellow fever vaccine.

Below: Freeze-dryer, as improved by Willard Webster in the early 1950s.

Bottom: Elmer Mader manufactures Japanese B encephalitis vaccine.

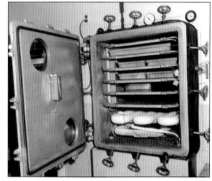

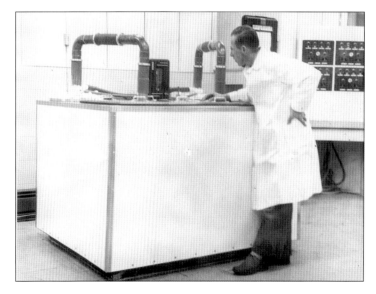

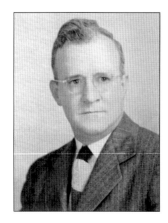

Another War

In 1950, North Korea returned the world to war. Once again, the need arose for vaccines for the armed forces, and once again, the people of Swiftwater rose to the occasion.

After World War II, National had decided to consolidate its operation in Philadelphia. The sudden jump in business made that impossible. During 1951, the gross sales of products produced at Swiftwater hit $2 million, greater than the sales in any of the war years.

"The space and facilities of our main biological manufacturing plant have become seriously overtaxed with the increased volume of business that our laboratories are being called upon to produce," the company bulletin, the *National Eagle,* reported. "This necessitated larger working areas and more modern facilities. To provide these necessities, a new building, connected to the present main manufacturing structure, has been erected and is now being equipped."

In 1951, National erected Building 7 for Biological Services and added to Building 3. The facility provided space for the production of bacterial media and media for the processing of virus products. It was also used as the site for the autoclaves, the pressurized, steam-heated vessels used for sterilizing equipment. The Anaerobic Unit, used to grow organisms that can live without oxygen, was also enlarged and modernized. That laboratory produced tetanus and gas-gangrene antitoxins, plus tetanus toxoid for human use, and for prophylactic use for the immunization of horses. The paper reported the production capacity of the laboratories would increase "by approximately 300%."

Above: Alfred B. Collins, president of National Drug, in May 1943.

Below: Aerial view of lower campus, 10 days before the Flood of '55 struck.

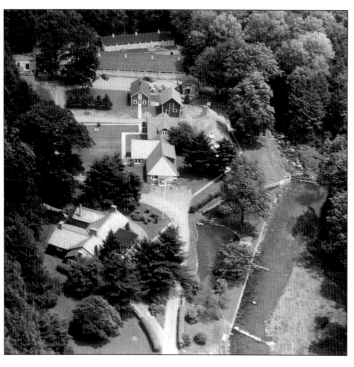

With the increase in horses to meet the increased activity, warehouse space diminished. To rectify that situation, National built a large Quonset hut to store materials. In 1952, Swiftwater become the sole American manufacturer of yellow fever vaccine and built a new isolation unit. Yet by early 1953, National president A. B. Collins was telling stockholders that net sales had dropped by $300,000 from 1951 to 1952. Net earnings had dropped from $309,422 to $295,000 during the same period. As Dr. Slee had done 50 years before, National was still relying heavily on government contracts. Apparently aware of that limitation, Collins issued a cautionary note: "It becomes more apparent each year that in order to maintain a successful competitive position in the pharmaceutical and biological markets, the company must rely on a creative and aggressive research department."

In 1953, the Korean conflict ended, and the Cold War began to rage. The U.S. government ordered large quantities of smallpox, DTP, and tetanus vaccines, to be produced and stored in Swiftwater in the event of a national emergency. A new tissue culture program was started, in anticipation of future production of vaccines designed to curb upper-respiratory infections caused by cold-associated viruses. The labs renovated the product-development building.

As for the Slee family, life went on despite the conflict. Prescott Warren Slee, son of Richard E. and Mary Slee and great-grandson of the founder, was born in June 1951, in Princeton, New Jersey.

The Flood of '55

If Swiftwater produced admirably during normal years, its people had a habit of performing small miracles during emergencies. They got another chance to prove themselves on August 18, when back-to-back hurricanes Connie and Diane dumped 8 inches of rain on Monroe County, causing the Swiftwater and every other major creek in the region to flood. On Route 611, the bridge over the Swiftwater Creek broke in half. At Camp Davis, a religious retreat in Analomink, bodies swirled in the wake. The flood contaminated drinking water.

Below: Raging waters from the Swiftwater Creek collapse the bridge carrying Route 611 in front of the labs.

Refrigerated trucks were brought in to assist local funeral homes. The storms left 99 people dead and caused $500 million in property damage in 13 states.

In Swiftwater, the laboratories sustained damage to many buildings as water and

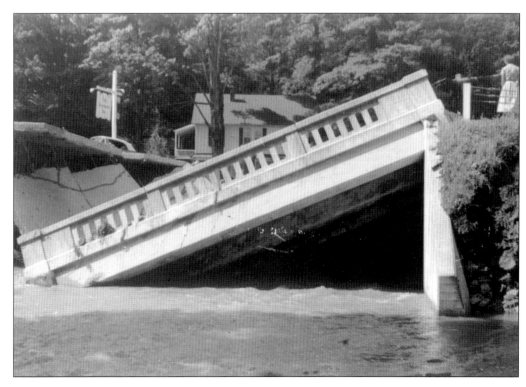

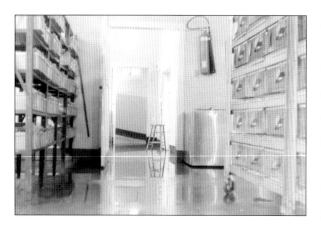

mud burst through walls and flowed over foundations. The blacktop roads and concrete paths winding through the property were eroded, leaving holes and impassable stretches. The lower pasture was inundated. Mud covered the floors. Trees lay against buildings. While water rushed through rooms, all animals and products were saved.

Despite impassable highways, workers made their way to the plant. Since the state had confiscated all earth-moving equipment, National brought a bulldozer and front-end loader from Philadelphia to remove the debris. "In a matter of hours, in what had been chaos, order was restored, and production once again established," the *National Eagle* reported that September.

Since Slee's time at the turn of the century, flooding had plagued the site. But it was not a natural disaster that would nearly put the labs down for the count. It was a man-made one.

Above: Water from the Swiftwater Creek floods the animal rooms, but workers sweep it clean of debris, and no animals are lost.

Below: National's Stenton Avenue, Philadelphia, location in July 1956.

The Vick/RMI Years (1956–77)

By 1956, the Vick Chemical Co. of New York, manufacturer of over-the-counter cold remedies, had decided to enter the biologicals industry. It targeted National Drug. In an article written for the local newspaper, Russell Knerr, then-director of the Biological Laboratories, said Vick chose Swiftwater because it offered "an available reservoir of labor and a geographical situation near heavily populated areas for reasons of economical and rapid product distribution." On February 27, 1956, Vick Chemical purchased National for $6.49 million in a stock transfer. National became a wholly owned subsidiary of Vick.

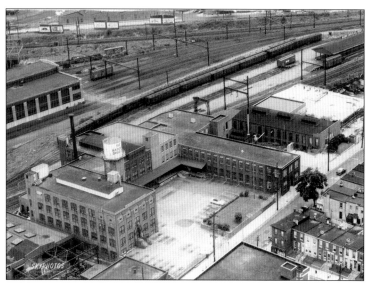

Even with new owners, Swiftwater continued to rely on government contracts. In 1957, approximately one-half of the output of the laboratory was supplied to the armed services, while the other half was sold to physicians and municipal, county, and state boards of health. That year, National Drug, along with four other manufacturers, received a contract for nearly 3 million units of Asiatic influenza vaccine from the U.S. Army. The first batch for civilian use — enough for 500,000 immunizations — was shipped by National that August. To meet the demand, National added another 50 people to its staff of 90. Webster led the Swiftwater laboratories in a crash program to produce the vaccine.

The effort was seen as vital to public health. In an editorial on August 13, the local newspaper, the *Daily Record*, noted, *"All these medical forces are coordinating their talents and efforts to provide us with a type of protection that was not possible during the flu outbreak of 1918–19, when more than 300,000 people died as a result of the disease."*

In spite of heavy rains that washed out 300 feet of shoulder on the road by the labs, the Swiftwater facility observed small victories. Employees celebrated the opening of its Ladies Lunch Room with a pork and sauerkraut dinner brought in by the women of the Appenzell Church. Alice Keiper's husband, Lloyd, captured the hunters' trophy for the year by killing a 350-pound black bear. Tom Hammil was the happy father of a boy.

Swiftwater's association with Vick continued to accrue benefits. Employees were allowed to save 1 week of their vacation for future use — a benefit that

Below: Map of the Swiftwater campus from May 1964.

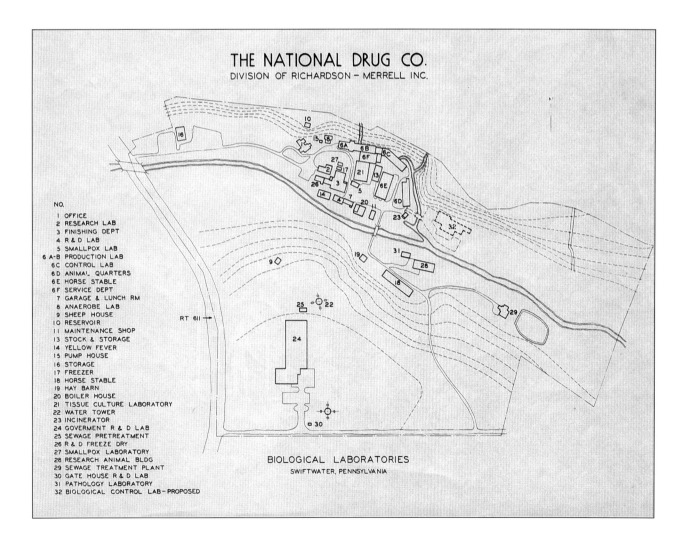

THE NATIONAL DRUG CO.
DIVISION OF RICHARDSON – MERRELL INC.

NO.
1 OFFICE
2 RESEARCH LAB
3 FINISHING DEPT
4 R & D LAB
5 SMALLPOX LAB
6 A-B PRODUCTION LAB
6C CONTROL LAB
6D ANIMAL QUARTERS
6E HORSE STABLE
6F SERVICE DEPT
7 GARAGE & LUNCH RM
8 ANAEROBE LAB
9 SHEEP HOUSE
10 RESERVOIR
11 MAINTENANCE SHOP
13 STOCK & STORAGE
14 YELLOW FEVER
15 PUMP HOUSE
16 STORAGE
17 FREEZER
18 HORSE STABLE
19 HAY BARN
20 BOILER HOUSE
21 TISSUE CULTURE LABORATORY
22 WATER TOWER
23 INCINERATOR
24 GOVERMENT R & D LAB
25 SEWAGE PRETREATMENT
26 R & D FREEZE DRY
27 SMALLPOX LABORATORY
28 RESEARCH ANIMAL BLDG
29 SEWAGE TREATMENT PLANT
30 GATE HOUSE R & D LAB
31 PATHOLOGY LABORATORY
32 BIOLOGICAL CONTROL LAB – PROPOSED

RT 611

BIOLOGICAL LABORATORIES
SWIFTWATER, PENNSYLVANIA

The Spirit of Swiftwater

was available, the company pointed out, in "only 2% of all companies."

By 1959, the future of the entire region looked bright. Direct-dial long-distance telephone service came to the Stroudsburg area. In a supplement to the *Daily Record* in Stroudsburg, the Pocono Mountains Chamber of Commerce described the region as offering the best of everything, including an "excellent geographic location, good labor relations, modern school system, outstanding recreational facilities, sound government, progressive banking institutions, and up-to-date shopping areas." Nearly 4,000 people worked in local industry with another 1,600 in retail for a total payroll of $24 million. There were 40,000 people in the Poconos, nearly 18,000 vehicles, and 687 farms. It appeared as if Vick had made the right decision.

By the end of the decade, the Swiftwater facility consisted of 21 buildings, two horse stables, a gasoline tank, and 40 acres of land with a market value of $469,102. At the time, the market value of an acre of land was $585.

Consolidation

In December 1960, the corporation changed its name to Richardson–Merrell Inc. (RMI). National was merged into RMI and operated as a division. National's injectable biochemical production was transferred from Philadelphia to Swiftwater. Two years later, Swiftwater took over injectables production from the Wm. S. Merrell Division of Vick in Cincinnati.

There were other changes. National obtained a 5-year contract with the sur-

Facing page: Barbara Bittner in Chemistry.

Facing page: From left, Harry Rementer, National vice president; Charles McCallister, National president; Russell Knerr, director of Biological Production; and Dr. Tony Bolyn, assistant director of biological production, break ground for Bldg. 21 in 1958.

Below: The Swiftwater Christmas party in 1959.

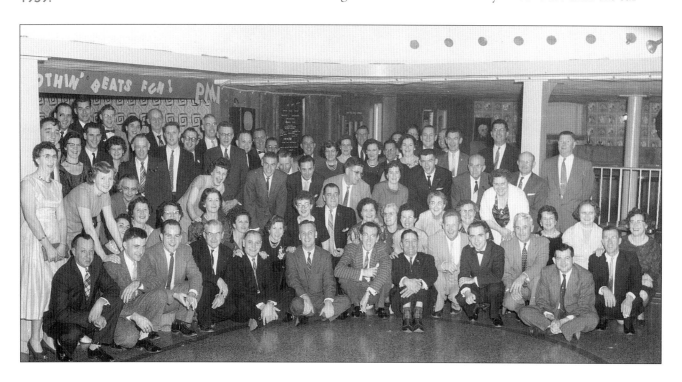

48

geon general's office to design a facility with isolated units for the development of vaccines against diseases that were not produced in the United States, and to develop a mechanized means of handling the possible production of these vaccines in developing chicken embryos. The agreement resulted in the construction of Buildings 24 and 25, the $2.6 million Research Laboratory (now owned by the Salk Institute). It also led Swiftwater to develop equipment to handle the large quantities of embryos that are required to produce today's influenza vaccine. The machinery was designed and built at Swiftwater and Stenton Avenue from 1962 to 1972, with the Swiftwater labs holding patents on the harvesters and inoculators.

Barbara Bittner, a lab technician and employee since 1962, remembers those days as hectic. "We were in a huge flu program," she said. "We were working 6, 7 days a week. We were producing yellow fever and smallpox vaccines. We had horses then, producing tetanus antitoxins."

There were few specialists in those days. "At the time, you moved with the process; they didn't have people who worked strictly in the kitchen," she said. "As a group, you got your equipment ready; it was sterilized. You got changed and went into the labs. At the end of the day, you took all of your equipment back to the kitchen. We were involved in everything, including the paperwork. No matter what it was, you did it. Today, people are more specialized. Back then, you learned what it took to get the product into a vial."

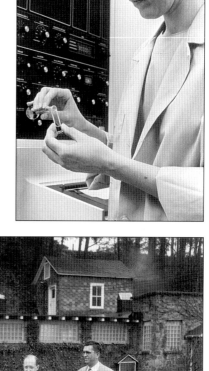

Even with the change to RMI, the National culture remained intact, Bittner said. "There were a lot of family members working here. They worked together. It was a major effort to get the product out the door. Today, you have a lot of teamwork, but the teams are within their departments. Back then, if it was flu season, the people rotated. You worked in the Filling department Friday, and on Monday, you were inoculating the eggs, harvesting the eggs, and batching the harvest. It was a great team effort."

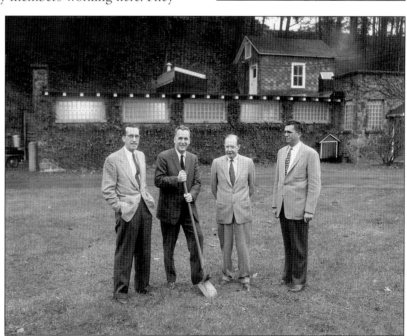

From 1961 until the middle of the decade, RMI would embark on a building campaign that would not always reflect its financial condition. In the year ended September 30, 1961, the new parent company earned $15.7 million before taxes on revenue of $42.8 million. In Swiftwater, it built the water tower emblazoned with the name National Drug Co. to provide automatic sprinkler systems with 100,000 gallons of water. It purchased 10 acres of land from J. Burton Hamblin and his wife to bring the total acreage at the site to 57.

In September 1963, National held dedication ceremonies for the Microbiological Research and Development Laboratories (the R&D building) at Swiftwater, which would later be turned over to the Salk Institute. In describing the facility, the *Medical Tribune* wrote: "The laboratory complex essentially is a one-story windowless building with perhaps as many built-in safety features as a nuclear submarine. Each of the four laboratory suites has its own air-conditioning system with filtration that has been proved against the passage of *Bacillus subtilis*. Intercoms flank every access door. Equipment moves in and out of the labs through giant steam autoclaves."

That year, National prepared to construct a 17,000-square-foot Biological Control Laboratory at Swiftwater, Building 32, later the Bolyn Building. It offered laboratories for in vitro testing, control test animals, and administrative offices. A mobile home was purchased to house the Pathology Laboratory, the first of the trailers on the lower campus by the Swiftwater Creek.

Results were mixed in 1963–64. While most products enjoyed increased sales, influenza vaccine did not do well, since there was no influenza threat or epidemic. Marketing came to the rescue, developing a 20-page coloring book called *Jimmy and Rosemary Get Their Shots*.

As for the Slee family, Arthur's wife, Phoebe, died in 1964 at the age of 78. Arthur then married Barbara

Below: Aerial view of campus in 1962 showing construction of Bldgs. 24 and 28.

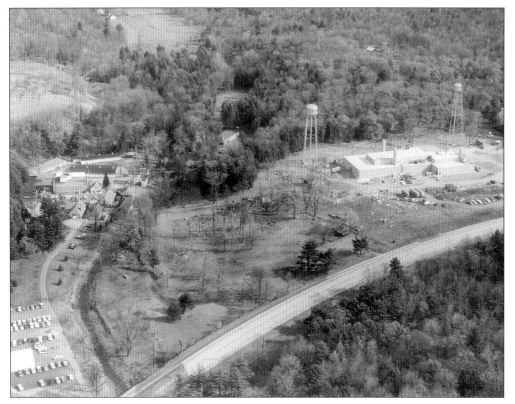

Edwards, the daughter of a prominent lawyer in Monroe County. His son, Richard E., who had been trained as a bacteriologist, and Richard's wife decided not to follow in the family's footsteps and entered the restaurant business in Princeton, New Jersey. Later, they put more distance between them and the company, leaving the states to manage a hotel in the Bahamas.

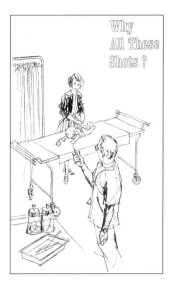

Preparing for Battle

The mid-1960s brought two changes to Swiftwater — new leadership and a new focus. One of the people who would lead the labs through their darkest times was Dr. Don Metzgar. The new focus, which would nearly scuttle the company, was flu.

In July 1966, Metzgar decided to leave Merck, where he had worked for the previous 5 years, and take a job as senior virologist at National Drug in Swiftwater. National had secured a contract with the National Institutes of Health Vaccine Development Branch to develop an adenovirus vaccine as well as parainfluenza vaccine. Dr. Joseph DeMeio headed the para program, Metzgar the adeno project.

Metzgar described his first visit to Swiftwater as a trip "through a sleepy rural country with almost no traffic."

Above: National Drug brochure from 1962.

Below: Aerial view of campus in 1964 showing Bldg. 24, the R&D labs, and the water towers.

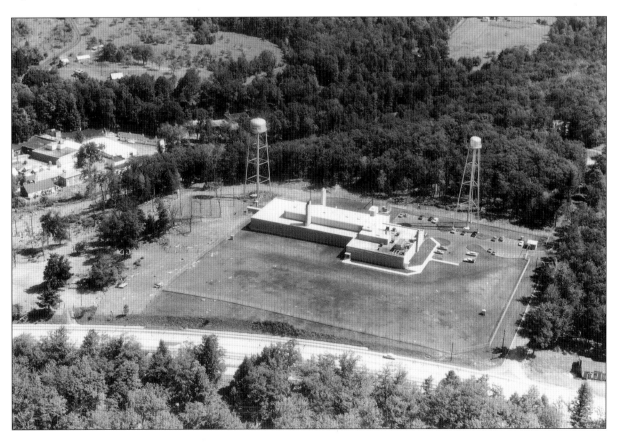

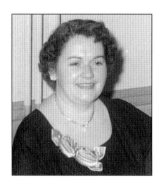

The landmark on Route 611 north that signaled I'd reached my destination was the water tower. I turned east into the plant area by the same route one hazards today. The difference is that there was no fence, no gate, and no gatehouse. As one exited Route 611, on the immediate left fronting Route 611 and Route 314 was a post office (the old Maginnis house), flanked on the south by a small American Legion memorial with a 40-mm cannon, a plaque, and a flagpole, where the Pasteur Mérieux Connaught sign and three flagpoles now reside. Immediately east of the house was a barn and stable with calves in residence.

The plant site was signaled by a Quonset hut with gas pumps and a small parking area on the east. There was no parking space on the south as we now see. Everyone parked inside the plant at their work area. Proceeding down the drive, I came to a small sign that said visitors with an arrow indicating one was to proceed to Building 1. My appointment was with Dr. DeMeio, and as I approached the steps to Building 1, a window opened and a woman stuck out her head and asked me what I wanted. She told me to take a seat.

Top: Ellen Regan, shown in this photo from 1959.

Below: Dr. Don Metzgar, pictured in the late 1980s.

That was Metzgar's introduction to Swiftwater, and Ellen Regan.

At the time, all product manufacturing was carried out in Buildings 6, 8, and 14. Volumes were small, as Metzgar recalled. "We produced about 2 million or 3 million doses of DTP, about 250,000 doses of smallpox, 500,000 doses of tetanus and tetanus diphtheria, 200,000 doses of bacterins, and 2 million to 3 million doses of influenza. Rabies and antitoxins were no more than 5,000 to 10,000 units. All of that worked out to about $3 million in sales, with a payroll of 132 people worth about $750,000." Bacterins were suspensions of inactivated bacteria used as vaccines. With no standards of potency and no proof that they worked, bacterins were removed from the market in 1972.

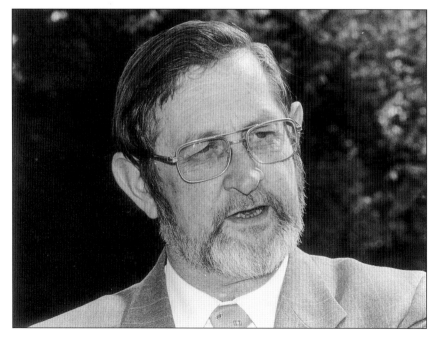

Antitoxins are animal serums containing antitoxins, used to prevent or treat diseases caused by the action of biological toxins, such as tetanus, botulism, and diphtheria.

Metzgar was soon joined by a man who would become a friend and fellow risk-taker at Swiftwater, lifting science to new heights. Dr. James Sorrentino left Walter Reed Army Institute of Research in August 1967 and went to work for National in Swiftwater as assistant manager of viral products. With key personnel in place, Swiftwater concentrated its efforts on producing a flu vaccine. In 1968, the company began planning for a new influenza facility, which would be later named for Willard Webster. Metzgar attributed the success of the program to forethought. "While the building was being planned, the equipment was being finalized and validated. It was an example where the facility was designed around a new and novel process. That is why the building has functioned so well over the last 25 years."

Things looked good. RMI sales in 1968 increased 12.6% over the previous year. For the first 9 months, sales for all of RMI's divisions totaled $226.2 million. By December, National had shipped 380,000 doses of monovalent Hong Kong influenza vaccine.

Then the cracks began to show. RMI began the consolidation of its two domestic ethical pharmaceutical divisions, the Wm. S. Merrell Co. of Cincinnati and National Drug. All biological research was to be carried out in Swiftwater. All other activity — management, finance, research, marketing, and sales — was to originate from the home office in Ohio. The split would not only cause immediate problems with communications but cripple the Swiftwater Labs a few years later.

For the Slee family, interest in the labs continued to dwindle. The descendants moved further from the site. In 1968, Deborah W. Slee, the great-grand-daughter of the founder, married Thomas Randolph Gibbs in Charlottesville,

Below: The changing of the guard, Sept. 24, 1962, when Russell Knerr, then director of the Swiftwater Labs, retired. Attending the luncheon were, from left: Dr. Joe DeMeio, Dr. Tom Granger, Willard Webster, Merlin Rutt, Dr. Harold Cox from Lederle, Russell Knerr, Ray Zorsi, George Prosser, the unidentified director of biological manufacturing from Lederle, and Dr. Tony Bolyn.

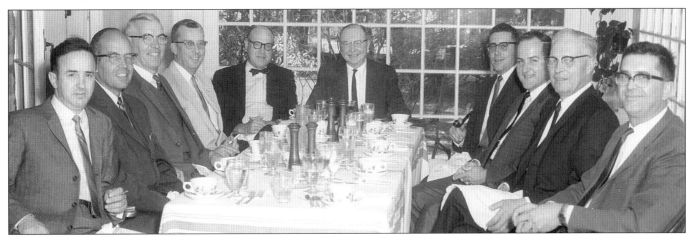

Virginia. Ten months later, her grandfather, Arthur, died in Stroudsburg at the age of 74. The Slees never returned to Swiftwater, except for a mysterious visit by Richard E. Slee. One day, the grandson of the founder was passing through the area and stopped at the office. A secretary called Willard Webster, plant engineer at the time, and announced Slee's presence. It took Webster a second to make the connection, but he walked quickly to the office to meet the man. Not quickly enough. He arrived a few minutes later to find Slee had vanished.

Hatching the Flu (1970–74)

After the merger of both ethical pharmaceutical divisions into Merrell–National Laboratories, RMI reorganized its biological division into a quasi-separate business and decided to make a significant investment in vaccines. Metzgar said the mood at Swiftwater changed overnight.

> There were great expectations on the part of the newly motivated Swiftwater operations. The government contracts were discontinued with the promise of an infusion of investment in research and product development designed to build the business and ensure the future. I was even promoted to section head and provided with my very own secretary, Marcia Bruno. Jim Sorrentino was promoted to director of Manufacturing and Development and, at last, given an office and a secretary as well — Mary Lynn [Vince] Argot.

When he took the job, Sorrentino was told to investigate a new influenza process. He now found himself in the position to do so. "The only problem," Metzgar recalled, "was that when he arrived on the scene, he had no lab worthy of the name. I had a lab with no money for materials." They worked out an arrangement that gave Sorrentino access to not only the lab but six extra hands, all with no payroll. Metzgar's team functioned as a serology and assay support center for Sorrentino's influenza vaccine development project.

The pair soon realized they could not increase flu vaccine production without automating the process. Eli Lilly had just published a pioneering paper on the adaptation of the ultra centrifuge, developed for gaseous diffusion enrichment of uranium by the Atomic Energy Commission, for the concentration and purification of virus — in particular, the influenza virus. The centrifuge would be used to purify virus from allantoic fluids, the embryonic liquid removed from eggs that have been inoculated with the flu virus.

Lilly lacked the automated egg-handling equipment support needed for such a system and abandoned the idea as workable but too expensive. Metzgar and Sorrentino embraced the concept. At National Drug, the U.S. Army program was providing data and equipment that suggested Swiftwater could handle up to 50,000 eggs a day.

Sorrentino ran into problems from the start. National did not want to invest the $250,000 needed to acquire the centrifuge until it knew the process would work. Sorrentino established a friendship with Dr. Norman Anderson, who is credited with adapting the centrifuge to handle biological agents, at Oak Ridge, Tennessee, where the centrifuges resided, and arranged to take the fluids there to be processed. Metzgar said the situation presented a logistical problem:

> How do you get a glass bottle containing 15 liters of virus-laden allantoic fluids from Swiftwater to Oak Ridge? Jim's solution was to rent two seats on an airplane and strap the bottle in one seat and himself in the other. The bottle was in an aluminum bucket. He would process the fluids at Oak Ridge and then return with the cuts and effluent samples by the same route. He did this four times that I remember. Once back in Swiftwater, we would assay the cuts and effluents and then he would be off to Walter Reed or Oak Ridge for electron microscope examination of the samples. This is how he built his data banks.

The vaccine was initially produced by concentrating the virus in the high-speed Sharples® centrifuge. The new process used the higher-speed K-2 centrifuge to band the virus in a sucrose gradient. The purified vaccine, Fluzone®, would be licensed on April 10, 1970.

In spite of Sorrentino's progress on the project, National's research administration decided the process would never be profitable and

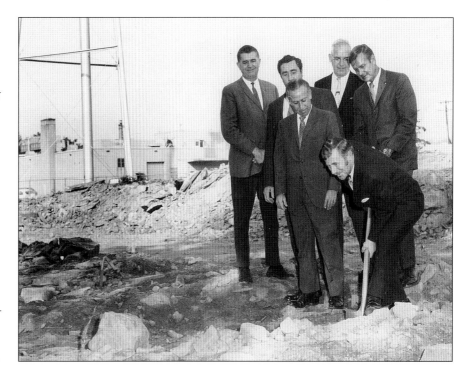

Below: Tony Bolyn, left, and Willard Webster, standing second from right, help break ground in 1970 for Bldg. 37, influenza production.

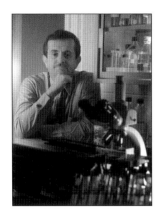

Top: Jim Sorrentino in his laboratory.

Below: Fred Capilupo at the electron microscope doing an assay on samples.

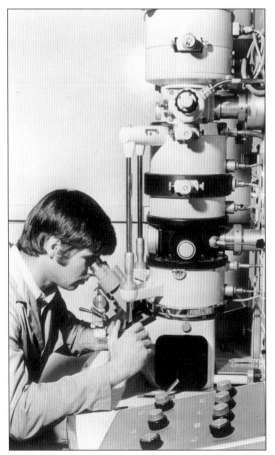

brought pressure on Manufacturing to abandon it. Research management put considerable pressure on Metzgar to deny research resources to the project. Sorrentino proved equally stubborn. He took his case directly to the RMI brass, president James Dodd and executive vice president James Gorigan, during a board meeting in New York. In 1968, less than one year after Sorrentino joined the labs, National bought its first K-2 centrifuge. It was installed in Building 6C.

Sorrentino's other contributions were numerous. He created several designs and modifications to the process that are used by the industry today. The reservoirs for the buffers and the sucrose solution were initially stainless steel tanks that cost $150 a piece. Sorrentino replaced them with $20 cans used to dispense cola at soda fountains. He replaced clamps and breakable glass connector tubes with quick disconnects made from stainless steel. His most important development was the console regulator, which controlled all of the fluids — buffers, sucrose, and allantoic — with the turn of a dial. It is used by the industry today.

In those early days of flu manufacture, Swiftwater consumed 10,000 eggs per day, 3 days a week, all of which were supplied by a local farmer, Elmer Veety. When the Webster building came on line in 1971, consumption soared to 50,000 eggs a day, seven days a week. It reached 75,000 eggs a day in 1972 and topped 100,000 eggs a day the following year.

The influenza manufacturing season began each January and lasted for 6 months. Its logistics inspired awe, even among employees. Upwards of 300,000 chickens produced close to 250,000 eggs a day, which were required to provide the facility with 150,000 fertile eggs of uniform size each day. They were incubated for 11 days and netted between 100,000 and 120,000 embryos for production. The cycle took place during some of the worst weeks in winter.

Sorrentino is credited with helping to create two breakthrough products at Swiftwater. The first was Fluzone. The second, in the early 1970s, was Menomune®, the first vaccine to protect against bacterial meningitis, which causes a disease of the meninges, the covering of the brain and spinal cord, and the first vaccine to use polysaccharide technology.

The problem in developing a vaccine was the large number of proteins in the bacterium, and the polysaccharide capsule coating the organism. If injected into humans, the polysaccharide would induce immunity against the bacterium, without the need for creating antibodies against a multitude of proteins within the bacterium. Based on a polymer of a sugar, the vaccine improved safety, since it only contained the polysaccharide and not the protein.

As with Fluzone, the vaccine was largely the result of the persistence of the entire workforce, especially Sorrentino. Metzgar recalled the Friday afternoon in 1970 when Sorrentino returned from a trip to Walter Reed with a 9-liter jug of *Neisseria meningitidis* Group C "paste" under his arm. "As he walked into the lab he shook it at me and announced, 'Metzgar, this is our next vaccine,' and so it was. The 'cookbook' consisted of handwritten notes and a mimeographed protocol from which reagents were prepared."

Immediately they ran into a problem — the lack of a key ingredient, sodium acetate, a reagent used in the process. "As I remember," Metzgar said, "we even called the East Stroudsburg State College, but to no avail." They finally found the reagent, and by the next morning, Sorrentino proudly displayed a 250-ml centrifuge bottle about half-full of a white precipitate. "Polysaccharide!" he proclaimed. It wasn't. It was still sodium acetate.

Sorrentino did not give up, nor did he notify management of the project until he had produced the first identifiable polysaccharide. The tactic worked. His credibility already established with Fluzone, Sorrentino received the support

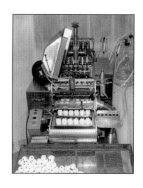

Above: Mark IIA egg harvester, used in the production of influenza vaccine in the early 1970s.

Below: This aerial view of the lower campus, taken in 1971, shows the Quonset hut, used as a warehouse.

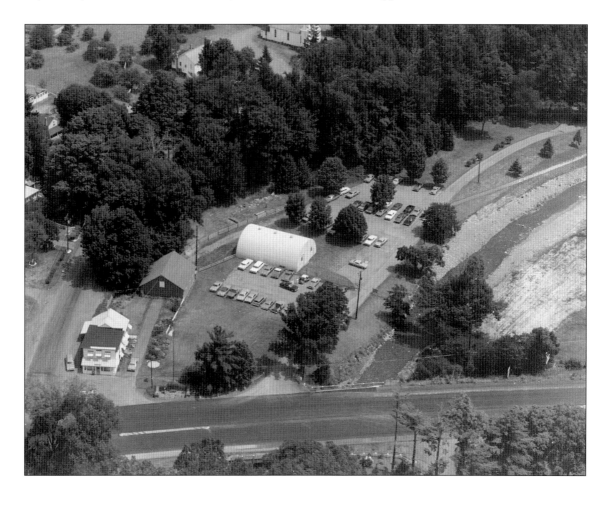

of National's management without much discussion. He also helped to secure the cooperation of a rival company. In an arrangement that foreshadowed today's emphasis on partnerships, National and Merck exchanged efficacy data via the National Institutes of Health and both were licensed for meningococcal vaccine, Group C, in 1974. National's product was named Menomune®.

Where Swiftwater would manufacture the product was a tougher problem. The market in the United States for Menomune was small — only for military personnel and travelers — and Swiftwater shared that market with Merck. There was, however, an international market. Institut Mérieux had furnished 120 million doses of Group C to Brazil, and the Sahal region of Africa was an endemic area. The solution was to renovate the north end of Building 9. Later, the bottles Sorrentino used were replaced with the glass fermenters of today.

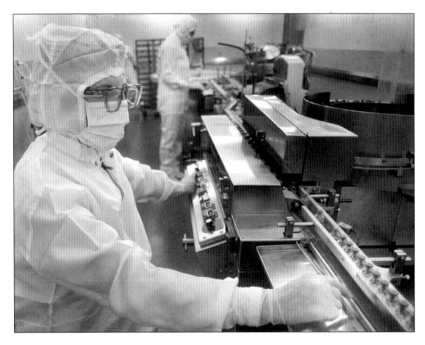

After Fluzone, Menomune was the second Swiftwater product to carry a trade name. It was the first polysaccharide vaccine licensed in the United States and the second one at Swiftwater to be lyophilized, or freeze-dried. The first was yellow fever vaccine.

In addition, Merrell–National Laboratories produced cholera vaccine, diphtheria antitoxin, diphtheria–tetanus–pertussis plain and adsorbed, gas gangrene polyvalent antitoxin, smallpox vaccine (fluid and freeze-dried), tetanus antitoxin, tetanus toxoid plain and adsorbed, tetanus and diphtheria toxoids adsorbed for adult use, diphtheria toxoid, and typhoid vaccine.

In 1972, Swiftwater turned once again to Pasteur Institute for collaboration. That year, Metzgar and Sorrentino went to Paris to obtain a new influenza production strain, then designated A/30C. In return, Swiftwater gave Pasteur the technology for influenza vaccine production. "We brought back the master seed and produced several lots for clinical trials, as well as 5 million doses of A/30C for Pasteur," Metzgar recalled.

Back home, flood waters again ravaged the laboratories in 1973, when the Swiftwater Creek tore through the lower campus, cascading over the loading dock and hurling rocks through windows. Employees were evacuated and seed cultures moved to higher ground. The Process Improvement and Development

Above: Workers use an automated system to fill product.

Lab, recently renovated, suffered severe damage to some of its highly sophisticated equipment.

The labs recovered, but bigger challenges arose. In 1974, Sorrentino left for a new job at Richardson–Merrell. Metzgar was appointed director of both Manufacturing and Research, replacing Carmine Mascoli. He implemented a cadre system of highly trained, interchangeable technicians who could handle every job in manufacturing and oversaw the development of new techniques and facilities.

The financial picture in Cincinnati reflected those innovations. By the middle of 1971, Richardson–Merrell's president, H. Robert Marschalk, reported that sales had reached a record high of $409 million, or 7.3% ahead of 1970. Earnings, however, totaled $32.5 million, up a little more than half a million dollars from 1969–70. "Our earnings were adversely affected by a lower incidence of colds than last year in the U.S and certain other countries," plus reductions in inventories, inflation, and a recession in the United States, he wrote. By mid-1973, RMI sales had increased to $446 million, then hit $556 million for fiscal 1973–74. The company employed 14,600 people at the time. All looked rosy. On the surface.

Dark Days (1975–77)

The world the Swiftwater Labs entered in the late 1970s was a turbulent one. President Richard Nixon resigned in 1974. The remaining Americans were airlifted out of Vietnam as war ended a year later. There were two assassination attempts on President Gerald Ford's life. The federal government bailed out financially ailing New York City. On a positive note, the nation celebrated its bicentennial.

Ford lost to Jimmy Carter in the 1976 elections, and the nation's economic and political climate became even more uncertain. Energy became a crisis. Iranians took Americans hostage. The United States agreed to relinquish the Panama Canal. On a personal level, life went on for the Slee family: Prescott Warren Slee, the great-grandson of the founder, married Michele Kathleen Burnett that June in Kalamazoo, Mich.

Things could not have been better at Swiftwater. The labs employed 120 people, occupied nearly 49 acres, and had a value of $2 million. In late 1975, the Bureau of Biologics of the Food and Drug Administration licensed RMI to manufacture and distribute meningococcal Group A and Group C polysaccharide vaccines. During the Vietnam war, the laboratories supplied tetanus toxoid adsorbed, tetanus and diphtheria toxoids, and diphtheria antitoxins to the military. It was, as Don Metzgar recalled, "a banner year. Everything went right."

In late 1975, the opportunity of a lifetime rose like the sun over Big Pocono mountain. An unusual A strain of influenza, swine–Hsw1, was isolated from sick military recruits at Fort Dix, New Jersey. The discovery would set off a public health hysteria felt around the world. It would also introduce the vaccine industry to a plague of a different sort — the liability crisis.

Even in the twentieth century, people reacted to flu outbreaks with fear. Since the 1500s, at least 31 influenza pandemics — worldwide epidemics — have been described. The most destructive epidemic of modern times, that of 1918, is estimated to have caused 20 million deaths, about 300,000 in the United States alone.

To head off a similar crisis, the federal government decided every person in the United States should receive a swine flu shot. The four American vaccine producers of the time — Parke–Davis, Merrell–National, Merck, and Wyeth — could not handle the demand. Production was delayed because the strain and reagents were not available until mid-March. "But the real road block," Metzgar recalled, "was the debate over who would be responsible for vaccine injury liability, since no carrier was willing to cover the risk, and no manufacturer would make the vaccine without the necessary risk coverage."

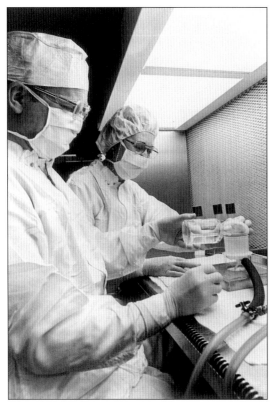

Below: Rodney Waltz, left, and Mabel Metzgar run tests.

Congress held hearings, President Ford declared an emergency, and the manufacturers, through the Pharmaceutical Manufacturers Association, offered to produce the vaccine at cost. In return, they asked the U.S. government to assume ownership of production, including liability. Congress agreed.

Under heightened security, the Swiftwater Labs built an entrance gate and guardhouse southwest of Building 1. It expanded production from 100,000 to 150,000 eggs per day, processing more than 44 million eggs that year. The operation ran around the clock. Centrifuge operations began at 4 A.M. and ran on 12- and 14-hour shifts. Two of the five centrifuges ran 24 hours a day. A second and third shift cleaned up the inoculators and harvesters on a rotating basis.

"The people at Swiftwater were dedicated to what amounted to a war effort," Metzgar said. "Everyone did their job. No one complained. There was a sense of accomplishment and celebration every time a lot of vaccine was completed."

The euphoria ended abruptly. Doctors reported an alleged

relationship between swine flu inoculations and Guillain–Barré syndrome — a relatively rare disease of unknown cause affecting the peripheral nervous system and characterized by flaccid paralysis — and lawyers discovered the vaccine industry. The national immunization program ground to a halt. The government had administered only 25 million of the 65 million doses produced; 15 million came from Swiftwater. The impact was quick. While Congress had assumed the liability by law, it took 10 years and a payoff of almost a billion dollars to settle the ensuing lawsuits. It took another 10 years to scientifically clear influenza immunization as a cause of the syndrome.

Vaccine-makers were caught in the crossfire. Businesses stopped offering flu shots, considering it cheaper to take the economic loss of illness rather than to risk legal action. The use of influenza vaccine dropped from 25–30 million doses annually to around 15 million doses a year.

The litigation was too much for Merrell–National. Publicly, RMI president John S. Scott was reporting solid financial results. For fiscal 1978, RMI sales and earnings per share reached record levels, with sales increasing since 1975 at a compound rate of 12.7%. Sales gains were led by products such as Vicks Formula 44 and Oil of Olay.

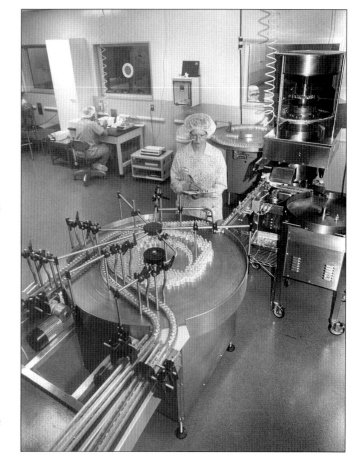

Below: Automation continues to play an important role in filling product.

Privately, the story was a sober one. RMI was not making money from vaccines. Swiftwater grossed $15 million in 1976. Out-of-pocket expenses related to the flu program amounted to $13 million. With the product liability issue absorbing more and more of management's time, RMI executives decided to leave the biologicals business.

The most serious impact was to follow. Swiftwater stopped producing swine flu in late November 1976 but was still finishing product in January 1977. Insurance coverage began to dry up and legal negotiations were time-consuming and tedious. Senior managers of Merrell–National were spending more than half of their time on a business segment that only amounted to about 5% of their revenues.

Early in 1977, Merrell–National Laboratories announced it would delay the manufacture of influenza vaccine for the 1977–78 year. Everyone at Swiftwater thought the move was temporary.

They made tetanus toxoid adsorbed and performed maintenance on the equipment and buildings. They also produced a large inventory of yellow fever bulk and meninge powders.

On April 1, RMI announced that it would divest the biological operations at Swiftwater and seek a suitable buyer. "This left us all pretty numb," Metzgar said. "Very little happened over the next 3 months. Representatives from Lederle and Sandoz toured the facilities but interest was cool. Others who might have had some interest were themselves considering how to get out of that portion of the business."

"The situation around here in the summer of 1977 was not good," said Willard Webster, who was plant engineer. "RMI had attempted to sell the biological laboratories unsuccessfully. They were looking for any way to get out."

Over the July 4 weekend, Metzgar found out what that meant. In a meeting with Howard Campbell, vice president of finance, Metzgar learned that RMI's effort to find a buyer had failed. "Rather than continue the operations, the decision had been made by RMI to close the Swiftwater operations by November 1, 1977," Metzgar said. "My role was to assist in drawing up the plans for layoffs and facility shut down. The only exception was yellow fever. At that time, there were about 154 employees, and the yellow fever plan would have left only 12. The trip home was one of the longest I have ever endured."

From July to November, Metzgar gave tours to representatives of Institut Mérieux, Pasteur Institute, Sandoz, Lederle, and Duphar, as well as Connaught and the Salk Institute. No one wanted the plant, so Metzgar, Sorrentino, and Jack Boyle, a former National financial officer, put together a plan to acquire the influenza and yellow fever operations. The plan was based upon Merrell–National providing a start-up loan and operating expenses for the first 2 years.

While the plan provided a compelling financial argument, RMI had a bigger concern — residual liability. In a scenario attributed to Howard Campbell, RMI decided to donate the Swiftwater Labs to a not-for-profit entity. That would negate the liability question, and the tax benefit would far outweigh the financial worth of the property had it been sold for the value of its real estate.

That October, the Salk Institute agreed in principle to accept the donation of the labs.

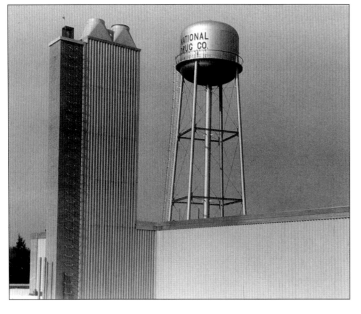

Below: In Swiftwater, National's water tower looms over the R&D building.

There was one drawback: If the institute maintained ownership of a manufacturing facility, it would jeopardize its not-for-profit status.

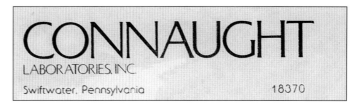

"In early August, Dr. Jonas Salk called Dr. R. J. Wilson, the honorary chairman of Connaught Laboratories Ltd. [CLL]," recalled Peter Campbell, then personnel director of Connaught in Toronto. "He said the institute had just gotten a call from Merrell–National. They wanted to donate the business but the institute couldn't take it because it was a not-for-profit institution."

Wilson, an expert in virology who had worked with Salk, considered the advantages. Connaught Laboratories Ltd. was at a crossroads in its history. It was supplying 95% of the vaccine requirements for Canada, a healthy nation of about 25 million people, but was locked out of the biggest market in the world, a few dozen miles to the south.

"The European market was fragmented at the time with their own state laboratories like CLL," said Campbell, referring to the Toronto company's status as a government-owned institution. At the time, Canada Development Corp. (CDC) Life Sciences controlled that country's major vaccines and blood derivatives producer, Connaught Laboratories Ltd. "We had maximized our share of the marketplace. There were restraints on the price you could have on vaccines."

Connaught sent a project team to Swiftwater for an inspection. "The deal was started in August and culminated at the stroke of midnight December 31st of that year," Campbell recalled.

In retrospect, the agreement seems logical. But at the time, some officials, including Alun Davies, president of Connaught Laboratories Ltd. in 1977, had some doubts.

> When I came to Canada in 1976 from the U.K., Connaught was in a devastated state, as was much of the biological industry. I asked at a strategic meeting, 'What is one of the biggest assets we have?' It was very clear to me the biggest asset was the world's largest market to the south. At this time, we were in the process of turning the parent company around. It was not making money.
>
> Our chairman, Dr. Bob Wilson, got a call from Jonas Salk about 6 to 8 months before the acquisition, saying that Merrell–National was thinking of dispensing of their interest in this field. They wanted to get out of a morass of possible legal

Above: Logo of Connaught Laboratories Inc.

situations. The company wasn't making money. They had developed a system that they could donate the labs to the Salk Institute, but who could Salk donate it to? With the antitrust laws at the time, the selling of the company to a U.S. company was going to be rather difficult. From a U.S. point of view, it was all risk and no gain. The best solution was to sell to a company outside the United States.

Davies flew to La Jolla, Calif., the headquarters of the Salk Institute, met with the principals and ran the numbers for Swiftwater. "We realized this company had never made that much money. We would have to restructure it so we could survive while we built a product line. It was a very complex deal. At the time, Connaught did not have a whole pile of money to invest. But it did have the desire and the expertise."

The Canadians paid the Salk Institute $1.99 million for 50 acres, including the commercial biological portion of the site. RMI then donated the 88,000-square-foot facility on the hill to the Salk Institute. (The Salk facility now develops and produces vaccines and diagnostic reagents for the U.S. Army.) The American division of the company would be called Connaught Laboratories Inc., or CLI. At the time, the transfer was believed to be the largest in Monroe County history, with the county valuing the facilities at $75 million.

Not everyone was enamored of the deal. Metzgar was concerned about ownership of CLL by the Canada Development Corp. and its implications. "I was provided with a copy of the charter of the CDC and was quite concerned that the opening preamble stated 'to provide jobs for Canadian citizens.' That of course would rule me out as well as everyone else."

Meanwhile, rank-and-file employees did not know what was happening. They saw strangers touring the facility and managers taking inventory. They were assigned busy work, or had no work at all, according to Dr. Ralph Vosdingh, who now works in Regulatory Affairs:

> I was in Research at that time. There would be groups coming through periodically but no one would say who they were or what they were doing. All kinds of rumors were flying around, that they were going to sell the company. The big worry was whether the new owners would keep us. Then a rumor started that they might just close the plant. There was not much production, but our research activities were still going on.

Then the word got out that the company was going to be donated to the Salk Institute, and Willard Webster's job was to take inventory for tax purposes. There was a lot of worry whether we'd have jobs or not.

The situation got worse with the rumor of Don Metzgar's list of who would stay and who would go. Vosdingh remembered the tension that rumor created:

> People started being interviewed by Don Metzgar. He had this little black book he kept in his pocket, and in this book he'd made a list of who was going to be discharged and who was going to get transferred and who was going to be kept and what their jobs were going to be. Mary Lynn [Argot] was his secretary. One day I got a call from Mary Lynn saying, "Dr. Metzgar wants to see you."
>
> He said something to the effect that the company was going to keep me as the veterinarian but that I would be transferred from Research to Quality Control and be in charge of the animal section. There were a number of people who moved up to Salk; some people were discharged, including the director of QC. I was disappointed that I wasn't going to be doing research anymore, but I was thankful I had a job.

Clair Wallingford, who had worked at National since 1938, said many workers found it a difficult time. "RMI didn't want us anymore. I was given menial jobs to do. I was determined to put in my time until 65. Here I had all of that training — I started the yellow fever program — and they started cutting people. That was a difficult time. You didn't know if you were going to be on that cut list. I ended up in the media department, peeling potatoes. The company was shopped around, and morale was low."

"Those were dark days," said Barbara Bittner. "They were taking inventory of everything that was in the buildings. We didn't know what was going on. The rumors started that we were going to be sold; the company was going to close. We actually had no work to do. We sat around and waited for the phone to ring. Then Connaught purchased the facility. One by one, they called people over to

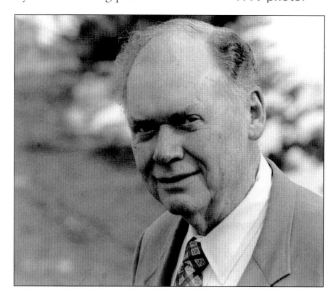

Below: Ralph Vosdingh in this 1997 photo.

65

Building 1 and you were told if you were terminated or going to stay on."

Connaught's Alun Davies said the payroll had to be trimmed from 150 to 110. Bittner, who was in Research at the time, was one of the lucky ones who kept her job.

"It was a very uncomfortable feeling to be kept on," she remembered. "It was hard to feel glad that they were keeping you when so many others were losing their jobs."

The mood in La Jolla on January 3, 1978, contrasted sharply with morale in Swiftwater.

"We flew out there with big suitcases of files to do the transfer from Richardson–Merrell to the Salk Institute, and then from Salk to Connaught" said Stroudsburg's Alex "Buzz" Bensinger, who represented the company that issued title insurance for both Salk and Connaught. It took one full day for the closing. "I never thought the Connaught transaction would be bigger than the Salk one, but it turned out that way. It took place in a small gymnasium on Salk's property, there were so many people involved. We sat at long tables, and

Below: Dr. Jonas Salk, left, and John Scott, president of RMI, at a December 1977 dinner at Pocono Manor Inn.

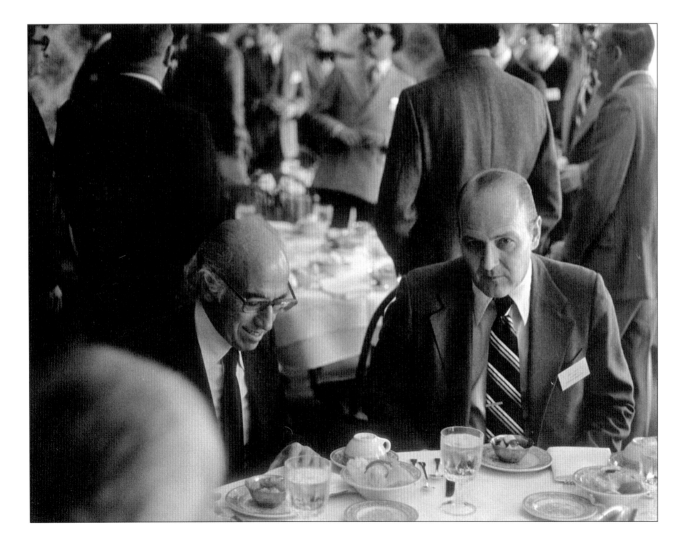

there were many documents passed around and changed and edited."

Bensinger had a personal stake in the transaction. Not only did he handle the estates of Richard E. and Phoebe Slee, but his father had done legal work for Dr. Richard Slee during the attorney's association with A. Mitchell Palmer.

Back in Swiftwater, there was little celebration. Willard Webster retired. There was no Christmas party that year.

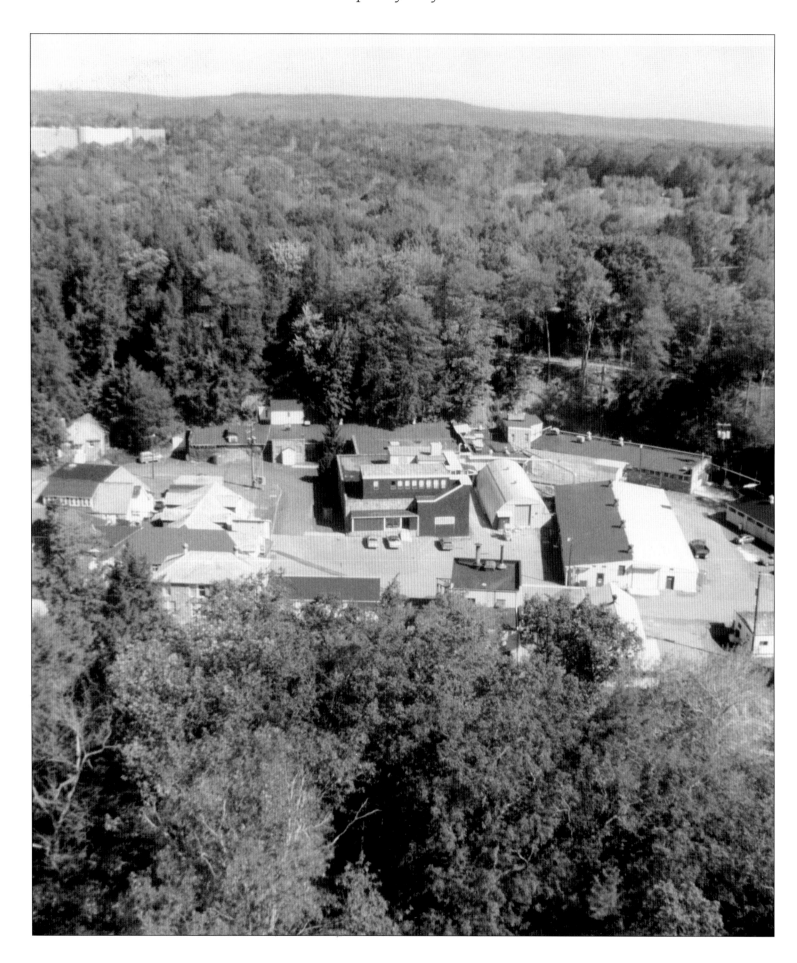

Modern Times

At the time Connaught entered the picture, the Swiftwater Labs were just one month away from becoming another tourist spot in the Poconos.

— Don Metzgar

A New Beginning

The Connaught Years (1978–89)

*I*t was cold and damp. Snow crystals hung in the air. On Peter Campbell's watch, the minute hand inched toward midnight. Soon the new year would arrive — January 1, 1978. The dawn of a new era, he wondered, or the end of his career?

Campbell had volunteered for this assignment, to become Connaught's first general manager at Swiftwater. He'd read the reports from Merrell–National about the labs, about a hard-working staff, and an aging plant. He'd seen the potential. He planned to create a highly autonomous operation, not second-guessed by Cincinnati or Toronto.

That night, before the papers were signed in sunny California, he stood by the lift gate, a single bar that would not prevent trespassers from entering, and stared at the collection of small stone buildings. The Swiftwater Creek bubbled. Rising from the hill, the influenza building and what would become the Salk Institute facility looked dark and empty. He noticed his heart was pounding.

He looked down at the little cottage that had once been the bachelor quarters and thought, *My God. Tomorrow morning, I'm going to sit down and people are going to ask, "Now what are we going to do?"*

In his head were the words of Connaught's board of directors: "You're going to make it work, but if you don't, don't expect to be welcomed back to your old job." He felt excited, rushed. Everything was happening so fast. Salk had to move quickly to retain its not-for-profit status. Connaught had to transfer licenses so that it could make products. He looked at the gate, thought about

Facing page: The Swiftwater campus in 1982.

69

the managers who had come before him. The employees had not seen much of them. He checked his watch. *These people think they get up early*, he thought. *I've got a surprise for them. I'm going to be there at six in the morning and leave at seven at night. I'm going to hug them in the morning and kiss them at night.*

Nearly 20 years later from his home near Toronto, Campbell recalled the challenge they faced:

> You couldn't just turn on a machine and start making vaccine. We had to determine if we could use existing inventory. We had new labels to print. And there were legal issues to resolve: If we finished product produced by Merrell–National and there was an adverse reaction, what do we do?
>
> We started the next day by cleaning up the facility. I said to Mary Lynn [Argot], "Let's get the files in order. Let's get out all this junk that had accumulated. Let's paint doors." One thing we were going to do was to keep busy. We were going to make this successful.

Below: Working long hours in the lab.

Transferring the licenses was the easy part. The real challenge lay in reinventing the company. All of the necessary infrastructure had to be built — finance,

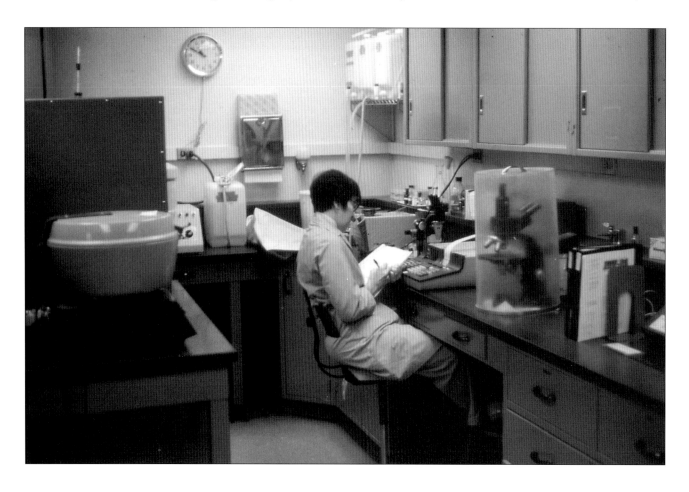

payroll, personnel, marketing, sales, distribution, and operating budgets. The let-terhead on all standard operating procedures, manufacturing documents, and protocols had to be changed to reflect the new owner. All of the labels, inserts, and cartons for product had to be reworked and reprinted. At the time, Swiftwater did not have computers, or word processors, to automate those tasks.

Adding to the problem was the condition of the plant. As Dr. Don Metzgar, who had been promoted to vice president of Operations, remembered:

> All of the facilities at Swiftwater, with the exception of Building
> 37, were old and in need of renovation or replacement. The tetanus
> facility was closed because it was unsuitable for further manufactur-
> ing. Building 32 [now the Bolyn Building, which houses Quality
> Control] was relatively new, but extensive renovations and updating
> were needed there as well, especially in equipment support.

The first draft of the corporate strategic plan placed a priority on replacing facilities at Swiftwater. Merrell–National helped, advancing Connaught $120,000 to construct a new tetanus building.

As if internal issues weren't challenge enough, the weather disrupted opera-tions from the beginning. That first January was one of the coldest on record, with one of the biggest snow storms in 20 years. For the first time in its history, the plant closed because of weather conditions. Stranded employees could not report to work, but the eggs had to be processed, and the animals had to be fed. As a result, those who could report were pressed into service where they were needed most. Some walked to work. Others stayed through the night.

That kind of effort from employees continued throughout the year. It had characterized the laboratories from day one and would make possible the suc-cess the company enjoys today.

The first product bearing the Connaught name was, fittingly enough, small-pox vaccine. Workers raced to produce, label, and ship the vaccine as quickly as possible, knowing that until the product went out, no money would come in.

Financially, times were tight. Even office supplies were in short supply. If workers wanted a new pencil, they had to produce the stub of the old one. Just as there was a shortage of supplies, there were not enough people to fill all of the jobs. As Barbara Bittner recalled:

> We had just been licensed for meninge A and C vaccine.
> Because the product was new, there was a push to meet the sales.

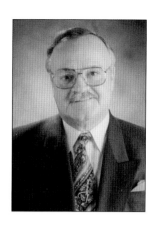

Above: Peter Campbell in a photo taken in 1994, the year he retired.

There weren't enough people here. There had been a number of people working in Chemistry who were let go after the Connaught purchase. I was brought down from Research to work in Chemistry. We didn't take our vacation after Connaught took us over. We sacrificed those things so the company could make a go of it. The workdays were long. We didn't take breaks. We would just work all day long. After so many weeks, I mustered up the courage to ask my boss, "When do you take time to go to the bathroom?" He laughed.

Campbell realized morale was sinking. "That first 6 months, people were saying, 'We're not putting anything out the door. We're going to fail.' I walked around the plant, I met and talked to people. I said we'll bring in 10 employees at a time and have sandwiches and I'll answer any questions I can. I ate more sandwiches that year."

The year ended with the acquisition of more trailers, the latest to house the financial operations, and another sign of growth. "The first-year plan was to have a sales volume of $5.1 million in U.S. dollars and an operating loss no greater than $150,000 to $200,000," Campbell said. "We ended up having sales of $5.2 million and a profit of $100,000. We went to a beer club and celebrated. I've had numerous celebrations since then on contracts that were greater, but none that were any more satisfying."

Below: Packaging for Vicogen®.

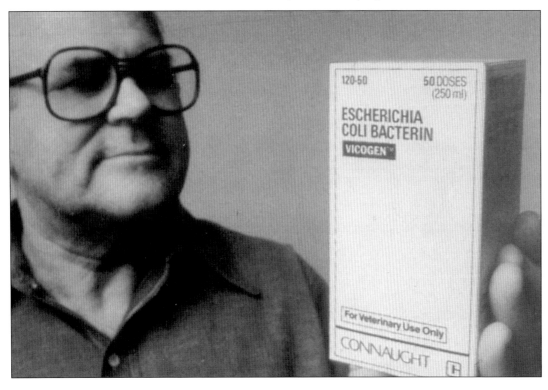

Despite the hard work, there were two more challenges that would test the Swiftwater Labs. One was the DTP scare of the 1980s. The other was called Vicogen®.

Two Steps Back

Veterinary products, which had been a staple of the company from day one, still played a role in the mid-1980s. Ralph Vosdingh, DVM, was the resident expert on the small but well-established line, manufactured at Swiftwater and sold by Pittman–Moore. Products at the time included vaccines for Eastern Equine Encephalomyelitis (EEE), Western Equine Encephalomyelitis (WEE), Venezuelan Equine Encephalomyelitis (VEE), and combination products. The company also made Tetnogen®, a tetanus toxoid vaccine primarily for use in horses; Inflogen®, a vaccine for equine influenza; and Inflogen–T®, a double antigen for equine influenza and tetanus.

Before it divested itself of the Swiftwater operation, Richardson–Merrell ran a veterinary business, Jensen-Salsbery Laboratories, from Kansas City. Swiftwater supplied tetanus bulk and manufactured equine influenza vaccine bulk for the subsidiary. In 1978, a market research study indicated that manufacturing a new product could allow Connaught to lead the U.S. veterinary market. The product, Vicogen®, was an *Escherichia coli* pilus-based vaccine to prevent calf scours.

This was the first veterinary vaccine developed from the pili, or hairlike structures, of the *E. coli* bacteria. As Vosdingh recalled:

> The USDA considered this the best vaccine it had ever seen for the prevention of calf scours caused by entero-pathogenic *E. coli*. Another innovative vaccine was a combination that included VEE, WEE, EEE, tetanus toxoid, and equine flu. This was the first such combination licensed by the USDA. All of these antigens were contained in a 1-ml dose. This along with the purity of the antigens and the unique adjuvant caused almost no reactions in horses.

Below: Profits were not on the horizon for Vicogen.

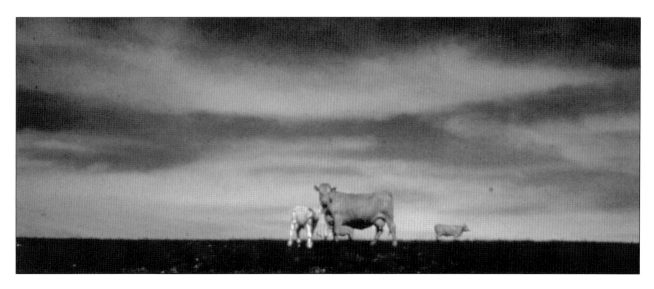

Pittman–Moore said that vets and horse owners called it the
Cadillac of equine vaccines.

Swiftwater first had to obtain a veterinary establishment license and a product license, which it did in an incredible 8 months, due to Vosdingh's hard work and contacts in the veterinary world. To meet the expected demand, Swiftwater modified Building 37, installed four centrifuges, and hired 27 people. Connaught set up headquarters for its new subsidiary in Kansas City, launched the venture with a press conference, and waited for the money to roll in.

It never did. Five million doses of Vicogen had been manufactured and 500,000 doses vialed in expectation of the launch demands. Crews stood by to meet the market needs, armed with a huge inventory of vials, labels, boxes, and shipping containers. The demand never materialized. Owners of large ranches did not want to round up their cattle for the injections. And smaller firms produced look-alike vaccines that cost less.

Metzgar recalled the disappointment:

> In that first year, we distributed about 120,000 doses of Vicogen, and a large part of that was either given away for promotion or returned unused. We turned off the lights on the water tower and the people that were hired with so much promise were let go. It was a huge let-down. Most people look back at this experiment with some nostalgic amusement, but what many don't realize is that the incident almost put Swiftwater down for the count. We had to absorb the losses, running more than $5 million, and it took more than 5 years to retire the debt.

Despite the difficulties, the year ended on a positive note. Connaught employees collected $1,096 for the United Way of Monroe County, a 71% increase over the $642 pledged in 1977. Swiftwater launched its first newsletter, called *Update*. And Ralph Vosdingh, who started with Merrell–National in 1975 to care for the animals and later to work on the *Haemophilus* project and Vicogen, was rewarded for his crash program with the USDA. In 1982, he was promoted to the position of responsible head, dealing with the FDA on human vaccine. Later he would serve as director of Quality Operations, which included Quality Assurance and Quality Control, then become director of Regulatory Affairs, Licensed Products.

Starting from Scratch

From the earliest days of the acquisition, Peter Campbell knew Swiftwater would never become a great company until it rebuilt the portions originally controlled by RMI from Cincinnati. To address that need, Swiftwater's first hire was a young accountant named Dave Williams.

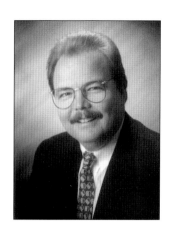

In hindsight, Campbell considered the hiring crucial to present-day success:

> One of the things I needed as vice president and general manager of Connaught was a strong finance group. We had the tactical people. We had the human resource person in Dan Gattone. But Finance and Engineering had been staffed in the head office. So we got this very young man from Coopers & Lybrand who didn't see the CPA [certified public accountant] license as his career path. He wanted to work in Operations. We held a couple of brief interviews with David Williams — what you see is what you get with David. He was willing to take a pretty high risk, but I guess he liked what he saw.

Williams had direct experience in the sales and financial side of the health care industry. Born in Scranton, he'd earned an accounting degree in 1973 from the University of Scranton and attended graduate school at night. During the day, he'd worked as a management trainee with American Cabinet, a small manufacturer of materials for multiunit dwellings. His greatest learning experience came when he was asked to supervise a small, contracted sales force. "These were people who didn't work for the company but sold our products. I had responsibility for their day-to-day activity. And that was a heck of a learning experience, because you were expected to deliver results without any direct control over the individuals — they were not employees. The experience gave me some foundation for my years here in Swiftwater."

He also had good credentials in the area of finance. After working with American Cabinet, he obtained his CPA certificate and accepted a job in upstate New York with Coopers & Lybrand, spending 5 years in Binghamton, first on the audit side of the business and then as a consultant to his company's health care clientele.

That combination of skills came in handy at Swiftwater. "He never was just the head finance guy," Campbell said. "He fulfilled the financial function but he was a member of the total team, in terms of bidding on products and resolving marketing and distribution problems."

Above: Dave Williams in a contemporary photo.

For Williams, the new company seemed like a start-up, which is one of the reasons he took the job. "The task we had before us," he said, "was to take an operation that was supported from a sales, marketing, and administrative standpoint from Cincinnati, Ohio, where Merrell–National headquarters were, and turn this into an operating facility overnight."

All administration, including payroll, had to be built from the ground up. At the time, the Swiftwater site could not market or ship its products in the United States. It could not even purchase raw materials.

Williams did not minimize the risk. "It is a fact that this facility could have met its end. Merrell–National, in those years, really let this place go. It was a manufacturing facility that was trying to become a company. They didn't have a way to pay people, purchase material, or sell product. I was young and foolish and figured if we could get a team going, we could make it. I felt I could get in on the ground floor."

At the same time, he did not exaggerate the challenge. The team — consisting of Campbell, Williams, Metzgar, Gattone, and Doug Reynolds, then director of Marketing and current vice president of Business Development — realized

Below: Bldg. 37, constructed in 1971 and later named for G. Willard Webster, became the main manufacturing facility for influenza vaccine.

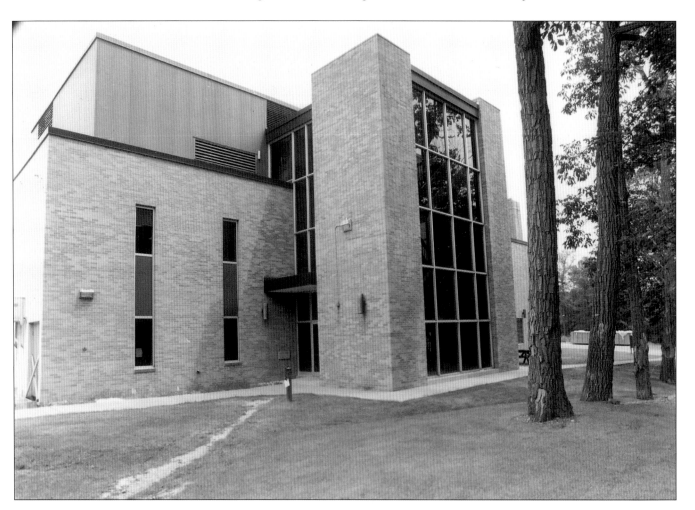

that while the risk was great, the opportunities were greater.

"Connaught was Canada's premier producer of vaccines," Williams said. "It was selling products throughout the world and sitting a few miles away from the largest market for vaccines, and it was looking for a strategy to enter the U.S. market. This was an excellent opportunity. The company had the ability to buy some bricks and mortar, pick up some products, and, virtually overnight, build an operating unit that in its first year had sales of about $5 million."

To provide a temporary distribution channel, Connaught had partnered with the firm of Elkin–Sinn for distribution in the United States. It also won 5 U.S. government contracts for 271,000 doses of influenza virus vaccine USP, monovalent A/USSR; 234,000 doses of meningococcal polysaccharide vaccine, Groups A/C; 1 million doses of yellow fever vaccine; and 207,000 doses of DTP. Connaught also shipped 1 million doses of meninge A/C vaccine to Nigeria in what was the largest single shipment ever made from Swiftwater to that country.

Buildings began to rise with profits, including the construction of a tetanus (anaerobe) facility. The company also began to tackle an old nemesis. Connaught officials testified at U.S. Senator Ted Kennedy's April 6, 1979, hearing on the government's proposed flu immunization programs for the elderly and chronically ill. Major areas of concern raised by Connaught, Wyeth, and Parke–Davis centered on the liability issue, and on manufacturers' risk in producing vaccine without assurance that such a program would be approved by Congress.

There were setbacks as well. In late 1979, Connaught did not win an $800,000 contract from the Centers for Disease Control and Prevention (CDC) for 2.4 million doses of flu vaccine. But the company rebounded with mass mailings of flyers to physicians and pharmacists, a move that became the de facto launch of a new strategy of direct-mail marketing. Times were still tight. That October, Connaught embarked on an energy-conservation project to insulate all piping on site. The project was expected to reduce fuel oil costs by $150,000 in 1980. But through it all, the employees persevered.

"The fact Swiftwater made a profit that first year was remarkable because it occurred in the face of obstacles that had turned many larger companies away from the vaccine market," Metzgar recalled. "A combination of liability problems, vaccine funding cutbacks, and public apathy — or even antipathy — toward vaccines had squeezed profits and exposed companies to more risk than most cared to handle."

By the end of the 1970s, Connaught had established itself as one of the leading producers of vaccines in the United States, if not the world. In 1979 it was one of only three world producers of yellow fever vaccines, one of four U.S. firms producing influenza vaccine, and one of only two U.S. firms producing meningococcal vaccine. The total product line had grown to more than 12. About 70% of Connaught's vaccines were used in U.S. hospitals, pharmacies, and physicians' offices. The other 30% were distributed internationally. The facility sported 15 buildings and 132 employees and used 120,000 eggs a day in the process of producing influenza vaccine.

Campbell, Williams, and the management team had done the arduous job of taking Swiftwater from the edge of collapse to profitability in less than a year. In 1981, when Campbell returned to Canada, Williams took the job of general manager. "When he left," Williams said, "Peter Campbell said to me, 'My job was to make this go. Your job is to make it grow.'"

Williams recalled the challenge. "The vaccine market, especially in 1978 when we entered the U.S. market, was categorized as a low-margin, almost service-oriented business with higher liability exposure than the larger companies' typical therapeutic products. At the time, we saw more companies exiting and fewer companies getting into the business. Of course, at Connaught, our business is vaccines, and everything we do is biologically based."

He had to play or fold, and folding was out of the question. Until the 1980s.

Crisis in the Courts

With a new decade came new challenges to the vaccine industry. Product liability suits, which had blossomed after the national swine flu program of the mid-1970s, multiplied again as parents and their attorneys alleged that DTP vaccines caused serious neurologic injuries. Pharmaceutical companies that also made biologicals dropped those product lines. "By 1983," Metzgar said, "there were only 4 serious commercial vaccine manufacturers left of the 12 that were around 10 years earlier. These included Connaught, Merck, Lederle, and Wyeth. Vaccines were low-margin products and, with the exception of Connaught, the pharmaceutical companies that had vaccine divisions treated them as little understood but vital public service enterprises."

By October 1983, the media began reporting on DTP, producing a TV documentary called "Vaccine Roulette" and a book entitled *DTP, a Shot in the Dark*. The publicity was followed by more than 300 lawsuits.

Metzgar said the vaccine and insurance industries were unprepared for the volume of injury suits that ensued. "Our medical and regulatory people were overwhelmed with the interrogatory demands for records and production information. Key people who should have been minding the shop were consumed with marathon depositions. Judges from a dozen different states were threatening us with contempt. Connaught, operationally speaking, was the new kid on the block, so you can imagine what the other producers were experiencing."

Faced with billions of dollars in potential litigation costs, insurance companies refused to cover vaccine producers, exposing manufacturers to risk and the prospect of bankruptcy. Pharmaceutical companies with lines of biological products, called "foster" companies, continued to abandon that segment of the business. Wyeth Laboratories halted production and sale of DTP vaccine. Lederle announced a self-insurance plan. Connaught had a more serious problem. "We could not get insurance coverage and we did not have the cash flow or the cash reserves to support a self-insurance plan," Williams said. "Since vaccines were our only business, we could not simply stop selling or producing."

In Toronto, Connaught executives, including Alun Davies, were concerned about their new investment:

> We realized we could not survive in business with lawsuits all over the place and prices that didn't meet the cost of production. At the time, DTP was selling for about $2 per 15-dose vial. That would not pay for the impending liability crisis, let alone fund research into new products.
>
> The whole U.S. market for DTP was about $5.5 million. It was clear there was no money in this business for anybody. I had tried to talk with competitors about a fund into which they would pay, but most of the firms were absolutely terrified of antitrust laws. A very senior official at a pharmaceutical company said, "How on earth can you stay in this business?" I replied, "You have a choice. You have other business. We have to make it work. The only way is somebody has to pay the price of leadership."

Below: Despite the DTP crisis, research and production continued at Swiftwater.

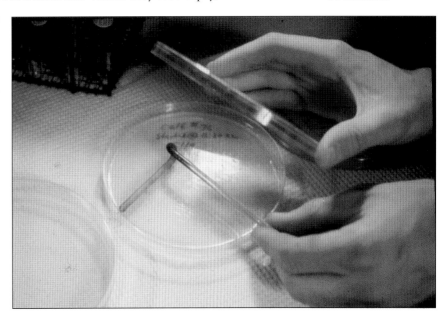

What happened next was considered crazy by many in the industry. Williams and Swiftwater's management proposed raising the price of DTP vaccine tenfold. Part of that price increase would establish a self-insurance fund to cover future legal claims. A portion, 15%, would fund the research of innovative products. As Williams recalled:

> This all started with the NBC special, "DTP Roulette," where they tried to draw attention to a study done in the U.K., linking the DTP vaccine to encephalopathy. [Encephalitis is any infectious disease of the human central nervous system characterized by inflammation of the brain.] Of course, history tells us that linkage isn't there. But back in the 1980s when this special ran, it created a stir. It created a situation where some parents who had children with encephalopathy for any number of reasons banded together and started to petition Congress to do something.
>
> There was pressure on the vaccine industry, too. It was facing billions of dollars in suits from a product where annual sales were measured in the millions of dollars. There was a disconnect. If there was going to be a continuation of sales, we had a new factor to manage, product liability, which until the time of the TV special didn't exist.

Despite the uncertainty, the management team knew Swiftwater had to act quickly. "One could view that price increase as a risk," Williams said. "We saw it another way. If no one else followed, the competition would get all the business and all the risk. If customers bought the product from us, the price would have the cost of managing product liability built in. For us, the real question was, 'What if we don't take the risk?'"

In 1983, Williams went to Connaught Laboratories Ltd. headquarters in Toronto to meet with its president, Alun Davies. As far as Williams was concerned, the future of the company was on the line, just as much as when RMI bailed out. During a joint conversation by phone with Doug

Below, from left: Hilde Gunther and Betty Leuber in the Filling department.

Facing page: Secretary Sylvia Lasher hard at work with the technology of the time, a typewriter and dictating machine.

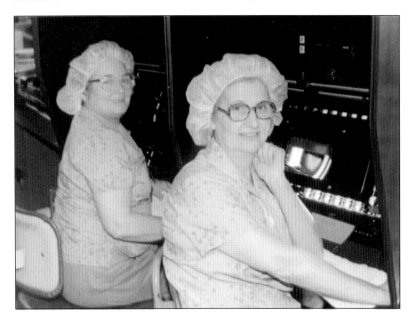

Reynolds, then-director of marketing, and Don Metzgar in Swiftwater's
Building 1, Williams summarized the issue:

"We can stand pat and hope the suits go away," he said. "If we're really serious
about building a vaccine enterprise in the United States, this is the right move
at this time. The status quo isn't an option."

Davies agreed. Yet despite the logic of the argument, the plan generated concern, both inside and outside the company.

Williams and his team stood firm. For a short time in 1984, Connaught
priced itself out of the market. Then, a DTP shortage developed. Lederle, which
continued to sell vaccine for 20 cents to 25 cents a dose, could not supply the
total market. Slowly, suppliers began to buy from Swiftwater, and other manufacturers raised their prices to achieve parity. "The competition didn't follow us
right away," Williams recalled. "We were alone for about 6 months. Then Lederle
also increased its prices. Wyeth eventually left the market."

"Soon we were at a competitive equivalence," Metzgar said. "We extended
the pricing and insurance policies to other products as well. The other producers
followed suit. The fiscal integrity of the industry was on the way to recovery."

The gamble not only managed the liability crisis but pumped much-needed
funding into research and development. In 1987–88, Connaught added four
major products: an influenza vaccine, Fluzone® split virion; an improved yellow
fever vaccine, YF-VAX® (ALV-free); a skin test for immune competence that it
licensed from Eli Lilly, MSTA®; and ProHIBiT®, the *Haemophilus influenzae* type
b (Hib) vaccine for meningitis and related childhood disease that became the
world's first licensed conjugate vaccine. The latter accounted for sales of approximately $40 million in 1988 alone.

Despite the fiscal solution to product liability, the lawsuits kept coming. So
did the price increases. Williams
said there was little choice:

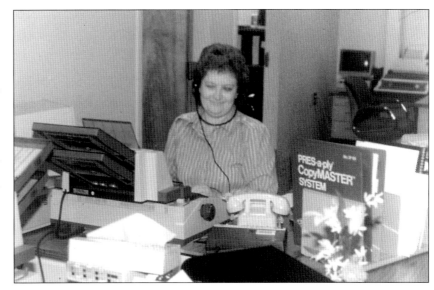

> The liability situation had
> the potential of destroying
> the vaccine industry at that
> time. The news media over-
> stated the rare reactions and
> did not talk about the level
> of disease that would exist
> without the vaccines. We
> had a backlash. We were

worried about the cost of dealing with litigation and the drain on management. Immunization is too important for the public health of this country not to take the proper step to fix the situation. The only avenue we had available was the price; we were trying to get the relationship of the price and the cost of doing business more in synch. We knew there was a level we could not go beyond without impacting immunization rates. Incremental solutions were not going to fix this problem. We turned to Washington for a solution.

As early as 1984, Williams began striving for long-term solutions, testifying before Congress a dozen times at hearings held by U.S. Senators Ted Kennedy and Paula Hawkins. On behalf of the entire biologicals industry, he initiated talks with U.S. Representative Henry Waxman to develop a bill that would be fair to claimants and manufacturers alike.

"What was envisioned at that time was some sort of a no-fault government solution," Williams said. "I argued for a three-pronged approach: swift compensation, just compensation, and an environment that fostered product innovation and supply."

Below: Map of lower plant in 1987. Building numbers have changed due to demolition and renumbering.

Facing page: Map of upper plant in 1987.

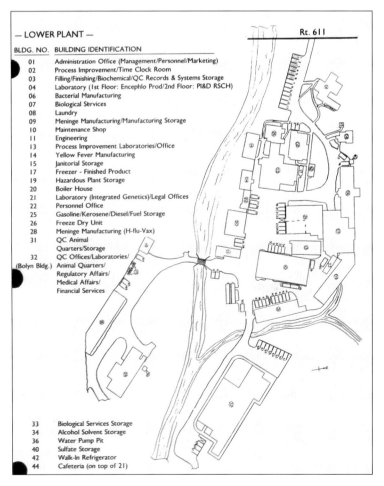

— LOWER PLANT —

BLDG. NO.	BUILDING IDENTIFICATION
01	Administration Office (Management/Personnel/Marketing)
02	Process Improvement/Time Clock Room
03	Filling/Finishing/Biochemical/QC Records & Systems Storage
04	Laboratory (1st Floor: Encephlo Prod/2nd Floor: PI&D RSCH)
06	Bacterial Manufacturing
07	Biological Services
08	Laundry
09	Meninge Manufacturing/Manufacturing Storage
10	Maintenance Shop
11	Engineering
13	Process Improvement Laboratories/Office
14	Yellow Fever Manufacturing
15	Janitorial Storage
17	Freezer - Finished Product
19	Hazardous Plant Storage
20	Boiler House
21	Laboratory (Integrated Genetics)/Legal Offices
22	Personnel Office
25	Gasoline/Kerosene/Diesel/Fuel Storage
26	Freeze Dry Unit
28	Meninge Manufacturing (H-flu-Vax)
31	QC Animal Quarters/Storage
32 (Bolyn Bldg.)	QC Offices/Laboratories/ Animal Quarters/ Regulatory Affairs/ Medical Affairs/ Financial Services
33	Biological Services Storage
34	Alcohol Solvent Storage
36	Water Pump Pit
40	Sulfate Storage
42	Walk-In Refrigerator
44	Cafeteria (on top of 21)

Rt. 611

Williams did more than argue. He created the Vaccine Policy Committee of the Pharmaceutical Manufacturers Association, now called the Pharmaceutical Research and Manufacturers of America (PhRMA), a committee he chairs to this day. He became the point person for most of the negotiations, including several postmidnight calls to Waxman. Williams and Swiftwater's attorney Carl Greco of Scranton wrote major portions of the bill.

Two years later, on November 14, 1986, Congress passed Public Law 99660. The National Childhood Vaccine Injury Compensation Act established a government standards defense for punitive damages in liability suits. To settle claims, Congress also created a no-fault fund, supported by an excise tax on pediatric vaccines.

"This was the key to resolving what was

rapidly becoming a legislative stalemate," Don Metzgar remembered. "Dave's work eliminated a serious impediment to the recovering health of the entire vaccine industry."

To this day, Williams keeps a miniature reproduction of the law in a Lucite cube by his desk. He did not get all he wanted from the bill: Despite its better-than-industry track record in liability settlements, Pasteur Mérieux Connaught contributes the same percentage of sales to the fund as other manufacturers. But Swiftwater managed to address the most vexing issue of the time. And just as Dr. Richard Slee had revolutionized American biologicals 89 years earlier, Dave Williams and his team had once again set the standard for the industry.

Taking Charge

While Swiftwater appeared ready to take informed risks, its partners were not. The labs still had no marketing, sales, or distribution capabilities. It had been working with the distributor for Canadian products in the United States, Elkin–Sinn in Cherry Hill, New Jersey. Toward the end of that 5-year agreement, Elkin–Sinn was acquired by A. H. Robins Co. It was a mixed blessing.

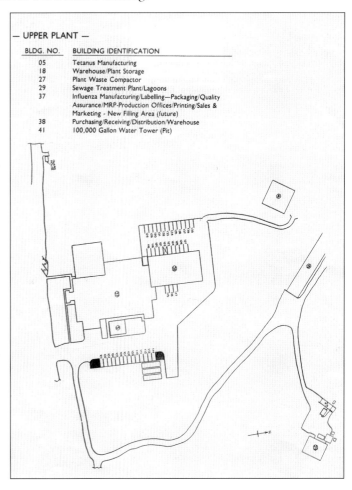

— UPPER PLANT —

BLDG. NO.	BUILDING IDENTIFICATION
05	Tetanus Manufacturing
18	Warehouse/Plant Storage
27	Plant Waste Compactor
29	Sewage Treatment Plant/Lagoons
37	Influenza Manufacturing/Labelling—Packaging/Quality Assurance/MRP-Production Offices/Printing/Sales & Marketing - New Filling Area (future)
38	Purchasing/Receiving/Distribution/Warehouse
41	100,000 Gallon Water Tower (Pit)

"We had access to a larger sales force," said Doug Reynolds, vice president of Business Development in Swiftwater. "The problem was, there were more than a few people within the Robins organization who didn't understand vaccines, and some were afraid of the liability exposure. We were looking for something more than a surface-deep distribution agreement. We were looking for a marketing partner. Robins wasn't interested. We started looking elsewhere. Through a contact Dave Williams had made with the people at E. R. Squibb & Sons, we established a jointly owned company called Squibb Connaught, headquartered in Princeton. That company was to be the marketing planning company for all the products marketed in the United States, utilizing the Squibb sales force and distribution network."

The company had its debut in January 1984, during the time litigation over DTP vaccines became a significant problem for the industry. "There was a substantial amount of anxiety about where this litigation was going to take us," recalled Reynolds, who was working for Squibb Connaught in 1984–85. "Squibb felt if the attorneys managed to bankrupt Connaught, they'd get into Squibb's pockets, too. Swiftwater did not have total commitment from the other party."

Swiftwater's leaders decided that if they wanted the job done right, they would have to do it themselves. "The DTP crisis gave us the opportunity to do something we'd wanted to do for long time — start our own sales and marketing organization," Williams said. "The dream had finally come true."

The decision allowed Swiftwater to become the fully integrated company it is today, with nearly 300 people in its sales organization and 40,000 customers.

The person who helped launch that force was Jim Brown, then Swiftwater's director of Sales and now vice president of that department. When he started on January 1, 1987, he had "one manager of sales training and one-and-a-half secretaries" in the home office. Sales the year before were $34 million. Brown hired six sales representatives, one division manager, and set aggressive budget goals, which his team then met or surpassed.

The company began making strides in other areas as well. In 1984, it became the successful bidder for the entire military contract for influenza vaccine, totaling nearly 3.3 million doses. The company also filled an order for more than 650,000 doses of the vaccine for the Province of Ontario, Canada.

The rest of the decade was marked by expansion and new sales records. That November, CDC Life Sciences Inc., a crown corporation that owned Connaught Laboratories Ltd. in Canada, granted approval for the construction of a $10.8 million biological manufacturing build-

Below: Ground-breaking for Bldg. 45 in 1987. From left: Dave Williams; Richard Schweiker, former U.S. senator; Bill Cochrane, chairman of the board of Connaught; and Alun Davies, president and CEO of Connaught Laboratories Ltd.

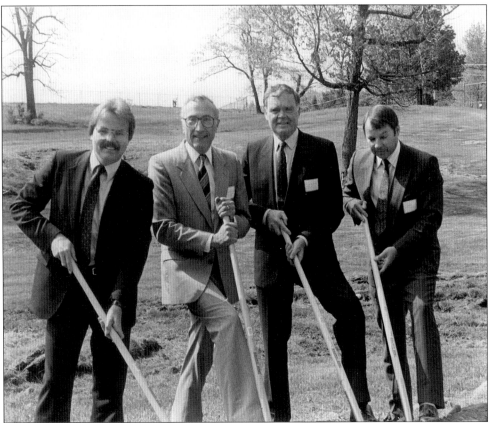

ing on the Swiftwater campus. At 31,400 square feet, Building 46 provided state-of-the-art accommodations for several existing products.

In May 1987, a groundbreaking ceremony was held for a $4 million, 35,000-square-foot administrative office facility, Building 45. In his remarks, Williams traced the growth of the Swiftwater site from 1978, with 110 employees and sales of just over $5 million, to 1987, with nearly 400 employees, a payroll of more than $10 million, and sales of U.S. $75.2 million.

In hindsight, it all looks so simple, the growth so inevitable. But according to Alun Davies and others who lived through those start-up years, the future was not always certain.

"Did we have doubts?" Davies asked. "Every day. But our philosophy was very simple. This was our business. Connaught was a specialist in this field. It was not a question of would it work. We had to make it work."

The decade provided challenge and change for many people associated with the labs. Don Metzgar would get to participate in the unfolding drama from the north. In March 1982, he transferred to Canada for the first time as director of Vaccine Manufacturing and Development. He returned in July 1984 to find that Williams had held open his previous job as vice president of Operations.

As for the original family of innovators, the Slees saw the births of two great-grandchildren of the founder. Prescott and Michele Slee of Holland, Mich., became the parents of Katherine Waldron Slee and Prescott Edmunds Slee in

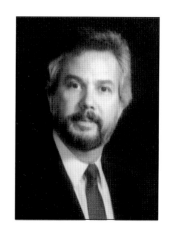

Above: Doug Reynolds in a contemporary photo.

Below: The structure of Bldg. 45 rises on a hill once occupied by horses.

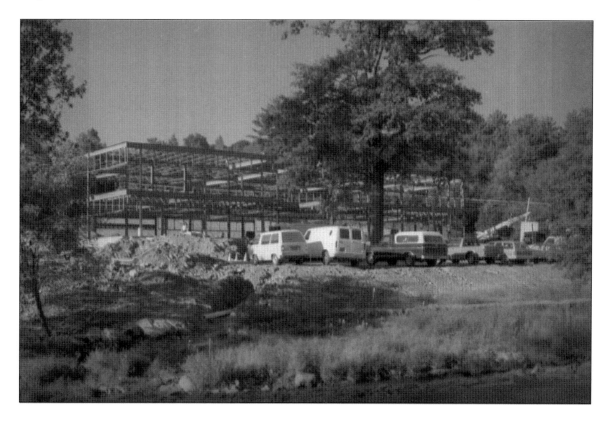

85

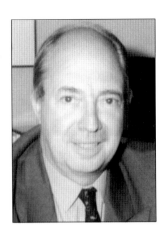

1981 and 1985, respectively. Two deaths in the family were also recorded that decade: Mary Waldron Slee died in 1984 in Richmond, Virginia, at the age of 66. Her husband, Richard Edmunds Slee, the founder's grandson, died in 1986, also in Richmond. In the 90 years since their ancestor had founded the Pocono Biological Laboratories, they had seen great strides in health care at Swiftwater. But they could not have imagined what would come next.

The Mérieux Acquisition

In 1989, George Bush was sworn in as president of the United States. The government bailed out savings and loan institutions and banned assault rifles. It declared war on drugs and invaded Panama to oust its leader, Manuel Noriega.

But the real action took place in Toronto.

About 3 years earlier, the management of Connaught Laboratories Ltd. realized that if they wanted to expand beyond North America, they would have to consider a merger with a worldwide company. They began to survey the field. Chiron Corp., a biotechnology company based in Emeryville, Calif., and Ciba–Geigy, the Basel, Switzerland, pharmaceutical concern, wanted to develop a vaccine business. The other major companies — SmithKline Beecham, Lederle, Merck, and Institut Mérieux — were strong in some geographic areas but did not cover the entire globe. That fact was not lost on the Rhône–Poulenc Group, which held an interest in Institut Mérieux.

Complicating matters was the status of Connaught. Owned by CDC BioSciences, a quasi-governmental organization, and affiliated with the University of Toronto, Connaught was considered a part of the Canadian heritage. To successfully integrate Connaught with a foreign company would take time and patience. To make the new company work would take someone with experience in merging cultures.

Georges Hibon held a unique position at the time. Currently chairman and CEO of Pasteur Mérieux Connaught North America, in the late 1970s he served as president of Merck Sharp & Dohme in France, Merck's largest pharmaceuticals subsidiary outside the United States, and, in the 1980s, as vice president of Merck International, based in Rahway, New Jersey. Hibon said with the backing of Rhône–Poulenc, Institut Mérieux realized it could successfully compete in a global market if it acquired Connaught.

"Institut Mérieux was very much focused on the Franco–Latino world — France, Belgium, Africa, and Latin America," he recalled. "The feeling was that Institut Mérieux needed to balance the company and achieve a strong presence

Above: Georges Hibon in his office in Toronto, 1997.

Facing page: Dona Reber at her desk in Quality Control.

in North America. Connaught had a good presence in the United States but little presence in Europe."

Alain Mérieux, then-president of Institut Mérieux, and his management group designed a strategy that included an exchange of stock. The French management then took a minor interest in CDC BioSciences. But the competition was also on the move, and Ciba–Geigy, which wanted to become a biologicals company, began its bid for those shares.

Negotiations were difficult at first, as Hibon related:

> The Canadians did not want to sell, especially to the French. They thought that Mérieux was interested in the U.S. market only. They saw Connaught as the only opportunity to have a worldwide Canadian pharmaceutical company. They said, "If we sell to the French, they have an organization in France and our role will be diminished. If we sell to Ciba–Geigy, they have no real vaccine organization, so Toronto will remain the central organization." With that in mind, we had to have a strong campaign.

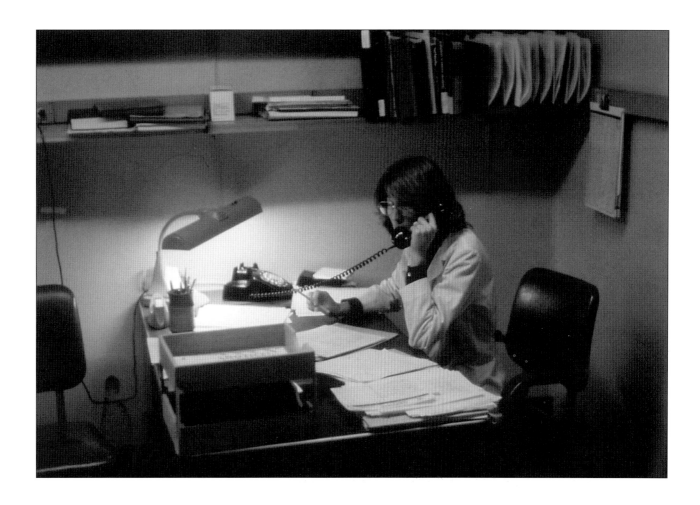

The stakes were high. "If you look at the vaccine market in general, at the time it was 40% in the United States, 40% in Europe, and 20% in the rest of the world," Hibon said. "As the cost of research escalates, you cannot amortize your expenses on one part of the world. It is important not only for in-line products but for future products. You need to have a larger potential market."

Ciba–Geigy had bid $31 per share. By November 17, Institut Mérieux bid $37 a share. On December 13, 1989, the Canadian government allowed the acquisition of Connaught BioSciences Inc. stock by Institut Mérieux, which paid $942 million in Canadian currency, or $781 million in American dollars, for the company.

Hibon, who joined Pasteur Mérieux Connaught shortly after the merger, said his biggest concern was the potential for a clash of cultures:

What I proposed was a soft merger. In my personal experience, I have been on the frontier of many cultures. When I was with Merck, I was sensitive to the differences in cultures. I said to Alain Mérieux, "You have different markets, people, and methods. You have to protect market share, minimize the impact on people, and use as much as possible the American methods." As a result, Peter Campbell and Dave Williams became part of the global management team with the ability to influence the non-American components of the company.

We got a lot of cross-fertilization from the merger. After the acquisition, we created five teams: Research, Manufacturing, Finance and Administration, Marketing, and Regulatory Affairs. We did not transfer a lot of people but we had a lot of people traveling. The early beneficiaries right after the acquisition were the airline companies.

Willard Webster, a consultant in the United States at the time, said before the sale, "People were holding their breath." Afterward, he said, life went smoothly at Swiftwater.

In 1989, the labs began a feasibility study to determine whether a

Below: From left, Micki Raymond, Pam Remey, and Mary Spolsky have lunch in a relaxed atmosphere.

Facing page: Mike Yacubosky between jobs.

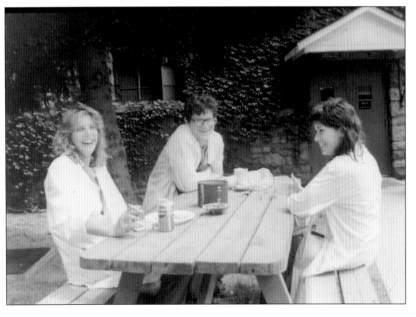

Lyme disease vaccine should be developed. Later that year, it expanded distribution of ProHIBiT® in Germany and landed a contract with the U.S. military for 261,000 doses of YF-VAX® yellow fever vaccine, which by this time had achieved a trademark. The Connaught Scholars program at East Stroudsburg University saw the donation of five $1,000 scholarships each year to biology and chemistry students. Alliances were formed to extend Swiftwater's reach, with Japan, the United Kingdom, Germany, and Iceland, among other areas. They were partnerships that would define the future.

So would a promotion at Swiftwater. That year, Dave Williams became president and chief operating officer of Connaught Laboratories Inc.

Partners and Allies

By 1989, the pediatric market had begun to change again, in a way that could have left Swiftwater behind. Doug Reynolds remembered months of planning when the concept of collaboration — combining forces and combining vaccines — was hatched:

> The strategic assessment about where the pediatric vaccine market was going showed hepatitis B vaccine, which had been used strictly for patients at high risk of exposure, was probably going to be recommended for routine use in children. The high-risk approach had been in place for 10 years in the United States, and there had been no reduction in the incidence of hepatitis B. If we were going to have a real impact, we had to make sure everyone was immunized. The problem was, they were already getting many shots, and physicians were saying, "How many times can I inject a child?" The idea was to develop a vaccine that would combine all these vaccines in one shot. If you were there first, you would capture a large market share, but if you came in second, you would lose the market share you already had.

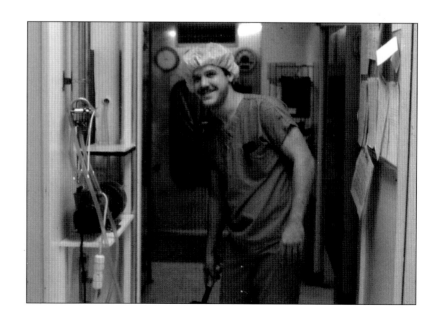

Shortly after the Mérieux acquisition, Swiftwater initiated discussions with Merck to develop and manufacture combination pediatric vaccines using products from both companies. "Merck had the hepatitis B but they did not have a DTP or polio vaccine," Reynolds said. "It was one of those things where neither one of us had all the pieces."

Spearheading those discussions were Alain Mérieux and former Merck International vice president Georges Hibon, who saw this as an opportunity to further their firms' global reach. "We looked at the evolution of the market and thought it would go toward a combination market. We did not have hepatitis B. Only two companies had worldwide rights to that, Merck and SmithKline. We started negotiating with both."

Talks with Merck yielded a limited partnership that focused on pediatric combinations for the U.S. market. The partnership was called MCM. Both companies would market the products. Hibon and the team now turned to Europe, negotiating a global sales and marketing joint venture for all of the European Community. The company, known as the PM–MSD (Pasteur Mérieux–Merck Sharp Dohme), was formed in 1991.

Williams said that set the stage for other cooperative ventures:

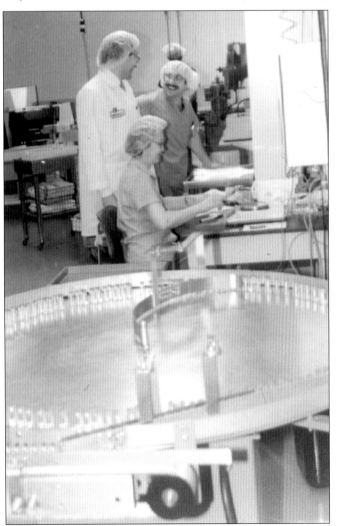

Below: Mike Macerollo, right, in the Filling department.

Partnerships have allowed us to develop combination products so we can compete in a complex pediatric marketplace. We are going to put together products that only one other competitor will be able to do, products that are going to play an important role in the public health environment. Partnerships will significantly enhance age-appropriate immunization, which is a problem in this country. Right now, you have acellular DTP, *Haemophilus* b, hepatitis B, and polio in four immunizations. We're putting those together in a single shot. It ensures you get all vaccines delivered at the same time, and eliminates a number of injections. Parents will be less troubled by the immunization process.

A key component that allowed the establishment of a combination product with all the important antigens involved the U.S. licensing of ActHIB®, a *Haemophilus* b conjugate vaccine originally developed in France by Pasteur Mérieux Connaught.

Strategic Shifts

Combination and conjugate vaccines were not the only innovations in Swiftwater during the 1990s. Pasteur Mérieux Connaught overhauled its marketing strategy to evolve with the economy. In 1991, the order-entry department, which began in 1985 with a staff of four as the company began direct sales of DTP vaccine, took on a new name, Customer Account Management, or CAM. Credit and collections and returns processing were integrated into the department. In 1992, a registered nurse medical staff was added; in 1994, customer accounts receivables; and in 1996, blanket order confirmations. The department now consists of 38 people, with the motto "One call gets all."

In sales, Jim Brown created a Telesales department that employed biological product associates, or BPAs. The program is unique in the industry and employs approximately 80 people.

Pasteur Mérieux Connaught also increased efforts to keep the community informed about its progress. It worked to integrate the new culture with the established one. And, to reflect its global reach, the company developed a new mission, Vision 2000, and adopted a new name.

Below: From left: Rose Kindrew, Colleen London, and Linda Petro. The early Customer Service department has grown to become a crucial component of the company's marketing strategy.

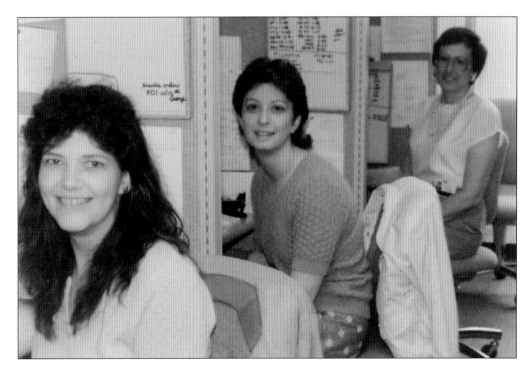

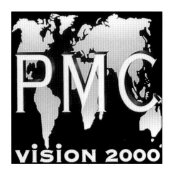

Evolution of Vaccines

Breakthrough with ProHIBiT®

As early as 1979, senior management at Swiftwater realized if they were going to compete in the market, they would have to differentiate the product line. Connaught carried too many generic vaccines indistinguishable from the competition. Innovation became the byword.

Doug Reynolds commissioned a market survey by Rutgers University that asked physicians if they would use a vaccine that prevented *Neisseria meningitidis.* They said no, but they would use one that prevented *Haemophilus* type b meningitis. As a result, Lance Gordon, who succeeded Ralph Vosdingh in Research, and Bill Hankins revived the work on *Haemophilus* b. Swiftwater already owned the rights to use the Eagan strain for research and development, purchased by Merrell–National in 1975 from Porter Anderson and David Smith, who later founded Praxis Biologicals. A second break came in the form of a paper by Schneerson and Robins, in which they described a procedure that would enhance the potency of a polysaccharide by conjugation with a suitable carrier protein. Conjugate vaccines use a fragment, called a hapten, of a disease organism attached to a carrier protein molecule to induce immunity.

Swiftwater went into clinical trials and the FDA licensed ProHIBiT, the world's first conjugate vaccine, in 1987 for use in 18-month-old children. The age would subsequently be lowered to 12 months.

"Within 2 years," Metzgar said, "*Haemophilus* meningitis almost disappeared as a childhood disease in the United States, and that included carrier rates." By 1996, vaccination had reduced the number of cases of the disease in the United States by 95%.

The development of ProHIBiT also gave Swiftwater a strategic advantage for the years to come. "When Connaught acquired the labs," Metzgar said, "it was a stated corporate policy that research and development was to be phased out of the Swiftwater operation and transferred to Toronto. The policy was never implemented because there was always a stream of new and promising products in development in Swiftwater."

Above: Pasteur
Mérieux Connaught
Vision 2000 logo.

Facing page:
Pasteur Mérieux
Connaught logo,
1997.

Race for Tripedia®

Concerned about systemic and local reactions allegedly associated with whole-cell pertussis-based vaccines, the company began developing Tripedia, a vaccine that mixed diphtheria and tetanus toxoids from Swiftwater with an acellular pertussis component. The problem was, early in the vaccine's development, the labs did not have an acellular component.

In 1987, the sales agent for a Japanese university group contacted Connaught Laboratories Inc. and suggested it incorporate a high-quality, acellular pertussis component in the American DTP vaccine. Don Metzgar, Alun Davies, and Keith Dorrington entered into negotiations, then called on the expertise of Walter Woods, director of Business Requirements Planning and Logistics at the time and now director of Project Management in Swiftwater. Woods and his team facilitated the project with the manufacturer of the component, the Research Foundation for Microbial Diseases of Osaka University, also known as Biken®. The Japanese were in the midst of an efficacy trial in Sweden, and Swiftwater saw the potential. Through its sales agent, Tanabe Seiyaku Co. Ltd., Biken sold the component to Swiftwater.

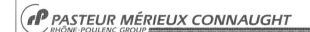

The acellular pertussis vaccine differs from whole-cell vaccine in that it contains only those parts of the pertussis bacterium that are believed to induce immunity against the disease. In clinical trials, compared to whole-cell pertussis vaccines, Tripedia produced fewer and milder local and systemic reactions.

That safety and effectiveness won approval by the U.S. Food and Drug Administration in 1992. The first license allowed Tripedia to be used for the fourth and fifth, or booster, doses of the DTP series. A second license was issued in July 1996 for Tripedia to be used in infants for the first four doses of the series — the first license of its kind for an acellular product. A third license, issued in September 1996, provided for the single injection of ActHIB combined with Tripedia by reconstitution for the fourth dose. A product license application for a single injection of ActHIB combined with Tripedia by reconstitution for the booster dose of both vaccines was approved by the FDA in September 1996, another first. That product is called TriHIBit™. At this writing, a license application for the use of TriHIBit in infants is awaiting FDA approval.

The use of ActHIB combined by reconstitution with Tripedia helps protect children aged 15 to 18 months against four diseases in a single injection.

As a footnote, the negotiations with Biken yielded another product for the Swiftwater portfolio, Japanese B encephalitis, a travelers' vaccine that Swiftwater now sells in North America, Europe, and most other countries outside Japan.

Eradication of Polio

In the late 1950s, microbiologist Albert Bruce Sabin developed an oral, live-virus vaccine against poliomyelitis. After field tests in 1957, it debuted in 1961 to become the most widely used polio vaccine in the United States, largely replacing the inactivated viral vaccine developed by Jonas Salk in 1952. (Salk worked with Swiftwater's Willard Webster in 1942 in the preparation of the first batch of influenza virus vaccine ever field-tested, which led Salk and his colleagues to develop the inactivated vaccine against polio.) By 1978, the wild polio virus had been eradicated in the United States, but 8 to 10 cases of polio resulted each year from the oral, live-virus vaccine itself.

In 1996, the issue came full-circle. Swiftwater had many ties with Salk over the years, as did Charles Mérieux, the son of the founder of Institut Mérieux. It also had access to a safer, inactivated form of the vaccine. Knowing it possessed a better vaccine, the company rallied support for a change in the vaccination schedule. In January 1997, the Advisory Committee for Immunization Practices of the Centers for Disease Control and Prevention (CDC) recommended that children should receive two doses of inactivated polio vaccine (IPV) followed by two doses of oral polio vaccine (OPV).

It was a landmark decision for Swiftwater, since the only manufacturer of IPV with an FDA license to distribute the product in the United States is Pasteur Mérieux Connaught. The product, called IPOL®, is manufactured by PMC at Marcy l'Etoile in France. If fully implemented, the CDC recommendation could increase demand for IPV to 8 million doses a year to meet the needs of the 4 million babies born annually in the United States.

Below: Brochures from 1993–94.

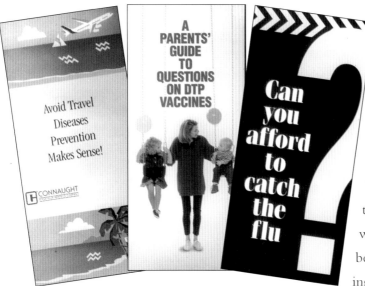

Evolution of Marketing

Long before President Bill Clinton started talking about health care reform, the marketplace had started to change. Managed care — a business model designed to limit rising medical costs — became a layer between the company that made vaccines and the doctor who administered them. Economics became a crucial component in deciding how health care would be administered, and to whom.

Swiftwater had the technology to produce innovative vaccines. Now it needed to tell the decision-makers about its evolution. And that meant a shift in its approach to marketing. As Dave Williams noted in 1996:

> If you go back to where we were 6 to 8 years ago, we decided
> the overall objective for the company was to be close to the cus-
> tomer, irrespective of managed care. We always have had a vision
> that our customer is the end-user who is delivering the vaccination.
> We wanted the customer to know us and value Pasteur Mérieux
> Connaught. So when managed care was coming into the fray, that
> put a middleman between us and the end-user.

Pasteur Mérieux Connaught decided to make systemic changes. As Williams noted years later:

> We looked at how we were organized as a company to address
> managed care, health care reform, and the changing health care
> landscape in the United States. We concluded that we had to find a
> way to work with managed care and continue the direct relation-
> ship with the physician.
>
> One unexpected variable was the fragmenting of the U.S. market.
> Ten years ago you could look at the market in the United States
> and say it's one market. Right now, there's a big difference from
> what is going on in California and in Pennsylvania and in Georgia.
> The first major change was going to a more regional area business
> unit concept, putting the capacity to change in the hands of the
> person who is running one of our regions.
>
> If you use the traditional model, which includes product market-
> ing, people focus on how to advertise and promote a product on a
> national basis. You have a common message, a common theme, a
> common approach. We recognize that things are different by region
> of the country.

In October 1994, Swiftwater reengineered its sales organization, creating business units to track and manage these micromarkets throughout the country. The charge to the sales force was to focus on the evolution of the market in their territories. Rather than having a blanket national policy, Swiftwater customized its approach to deal with the evolution occurring at specific locations. "Their job," Williams said of the business units, "is to understand these changes and to have the business plans to adapt to them."

Pasteur Mérieux Connaught also realized that with a shift in economics came a shift in perception, one that could have been detrimental to Swiftwater. Williams addressed the issue this way:

Two years ago, we had to realize that managed care doesn't care about vaccines. They do care about immunization rates. We are now partnering with the focus on improving immunization rates. If you talk about vaccines, managed care asks, "What's your price?" If you say, "We want to talk about your immunization rates, we want you to partner with us," you get a different response. Now we are a presence with managed care. In surveys that show how companies are perceived, we have gone from being nowhere to being on top. Success is measured by whether we're forming the relationships, and we are.

Evolution of Culture

There are other relationships, internal ones, that Swiftwater is trying to bolster. As Pasteur Mérieux Connaught integrates numerous groups through acquisition, as it continues to grow with new markets and new workers, it faces some concerns about a confluence of cultures.

On a day when Swiftwater-based employees received a landmark check from the state of Pennsylvania, the company's sales force held a launch rally for Tripedia in Texas. As young workers donned headsets and mounted a telemarketing campaign, the Twenty Year Club celebrated its fiftieth

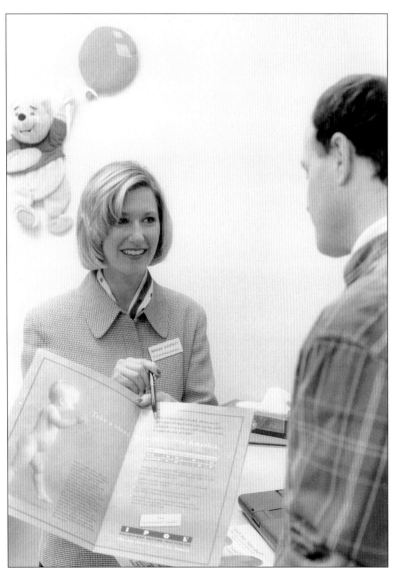

Below: Monique Cleverley, biological products specialist, discusses IPOL® with a doctor in Allentown, Pennsylvania, in 1997.

anniversary with a talk on history by Willard Webster.

Barbara Bittner, who has worked for the company since 1962 and now serves on both picnic and community relations committees, sees established and emerging cultures complementing each other:

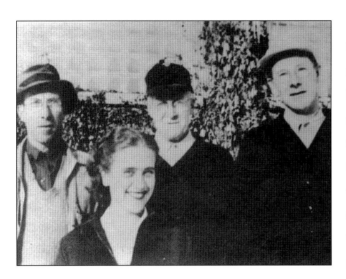

> What I like about Swiftwater today is the atmosphere and the culture. It is still the same company, just bigger. A few years ago, upper management wanted to incorporate older culture with the newer culture. If you look at the anniversaries, there is a big difference — 30 years and 5 years. How could they bring the two cultures together? They defined the old culture, like the company outing, and worked to blend both cultures. You see these people every day and you know their faces, you just don't know the names. The new employees want these family get-togethers, too.

One thing that has not changed is Swiftwater's commitment to the community. In 1992, the Employees Club collected food, water, and money for Floridians affected by Hurricane Andrew. The year before, Swiftwater made a record donation of $52,000 to the United Way of Monroe County, making Pasteur Mérieux Connaught the largest contributor to the non-profit organization. Employees surpassed that goal in 1992, raising more than $60,000, and topped it again in 1994 with a contribution of $65,000. In 1995, employees raised more than $90,000 — the single largest donation in the history of the campaign. In 1996, the number soared past $100,000 to account for more than one-eighth of the entire United Way of Monroe County budget.

"The old culture," Bittner said, "was that the employees were very active in their communities, through walk-a-thons and other activities. In the new cul-

Left: The Mader family worked at Swiftwater Biological Laboratories for decades: From left, Elmer, Gloria, Charles ('Pop'), and Clarence ('Jackie'). Charles joined National Drug in 1927; Clarence, his son, in 1928; Elmer in 1929; and Gloria, daughter of Elmer and Elsie, in 1950.

Below: Barbara Bittner, Quality Control/Chemistry, in 1997.

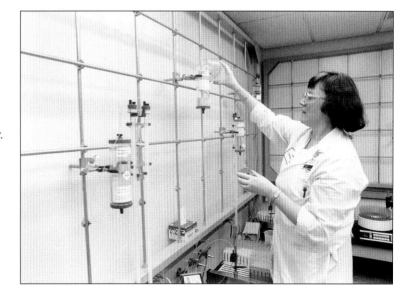

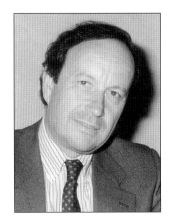

ture, the company supports its employees' involvement in the community. We want the community to know we give something back.

"I think we have a great blend of both cultures."

Evolution of the Name

With the changing of the guard came a change in name. In 1911, the Pocono Biological Laboratories became the Slee Laboratories. Swiftwater became the National Drug Co. when it was leased by National in 1927. It retained the name when Vick Chemical Co. acquired the company in 1956 and when Richardson–Merrell Inc. (RMI) acquired National in 1961.

Another change occurred in 1971, when RMI consolidated its two domestic ethical pharmaceutical divisions, National Drug and the Wm. S. Merrell Co. The new company was called Merrell–National Laboratories and retained that name until 1978, when Connaught Laboratories Ltd. purchased the firm and renamed the American operation Connaught Laboratories Inc.

The name held through the 1989 acquisition of Connaught by Institut Mérieux S.A. but gave way in 1996 to a more unified corporate identity. That November, Connaught Laboratories Inc. became known as Pasteur Mérieux Connaught, with a new logo and a consolidated global identity to better reflect the company's combined strength, heritage, and status as a member of the Rhône–Poulenc Group. The new identity is shared by Pasteur Mérieux Serums & Vaccines S.A. of France, Connaught Laboratories Ltd. of Canada, and the Swiftwater Labs — all a part of the parent company, Rhône–Poulenc S.A.

Above: Jean-Jacques Bertrand in his office, 1997.

Below: Pennsylvania Gov. Tom Ridge mingles with the crowd at Swiftwater after presenting a check for $1 million.

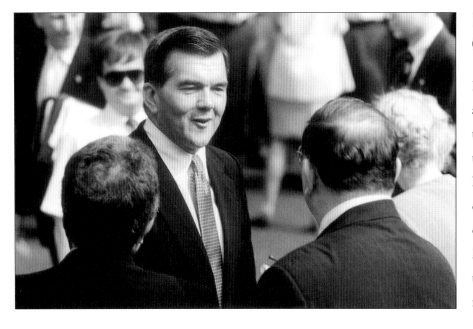

Breaking New Ground

It was a bright, warm day — a sharp contrast to the conditions Peter Campbell faced that icy night when he took his midnight stroll to the company gate. Some 300 employees of Pasteur Mérieux Connaught lined the parking lot in front of the main administration building in Swiftwater to listen to Pennsylvania Governor Tom Ridge and PMC USA president Dave Williams talk about new partners and new opportunities for growth. There was another contrast with that bleak night 19 years ago: The governor was holding a check for $1 million.

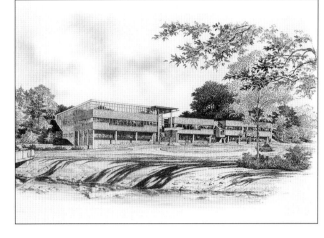

That summer day in 1996 was a first for Swiftwater, and the community: the first time the governor of Pennsylvania had paid a visit to the campus, and the first time the Commonwealth had offered a grant from its new Opportunity Fund, a $25-million initiative designed to keep jobs in the state. It was also a tremendous achievement for

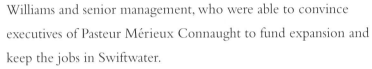

Williams and senior management, who were able to convince executives of Pasteur Mérieux Connaught to fund expansion and keep the jobs in Swiftwater.

"This is a company that has resources to locate anywhere in the world," Ridge acknowledged. "We think [the grant] is a great investment in our community. Biotechnology holds amazing promise as the growth industry for the next century, and I want to make Pennsylvania a leader in that movement."

The grant supported a $9-million expansion project at Swiftwater that included new personnel, training, equipment, and an 87,500-square-foot addition to Building 45, called Building 50. The funding will help ensure the retention of jobs and the creation of new ones in Swiftwater. In addition to the $1 million grant, the Ridge Administration approved a $1 million low-interest loan from the Pennsylvania Industrial Development Authority to help fund the Swiftwater capital investment program over the next 5 years.

Ridge spent the morning at the Swiftwater site, first meeting with senior management, then touring the facilities and helping to conduct an experiment involving a test that detects antibody binding interactions. He then spoke with an employee from the governor's hometown of Erie, Pennsylvania, who presented

Above: Artist's rendering of Bldg. 50.

Left: Dave Williams, president of Pasteur Mérieux Connaught USA, leads groundbreaking ceremony.

Below: After the ceremony, employees enjoy lunch under the tents.

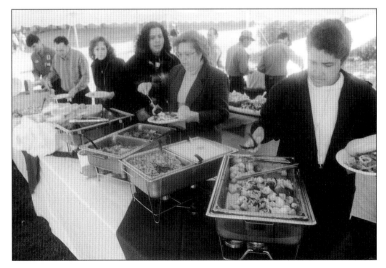

The Spirit of Swiftwater

him with the front page of the *Erie Daily Times*. The paper announced the FDA licensing of Tripedia for use in infants, the first vaccine of its kind to be granted a license in the United States.

It was a groundbreaking occasion. But the real earth-moving would come three-and-a-half months later.

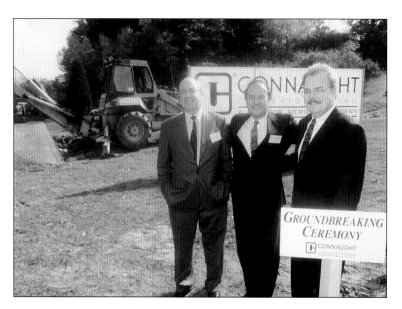

Building Recognition

It was another warm, sunny day in October as employees and dignitaries once again gathered in front of the administration building, this time to celebrate the groundbreaking for the new addition. A stage stood on the spot where a structure three times the size of Building 45 would rise. Tents and picnic tables dotted the lawn where employees would soon share lunch and discuss the future.

This time, instead of Tom Ridge and his entourage, Dave Williams presided over a group that included Georges Hibon, chairman and CEO of Pasteur Mérieux Connaught North America; Jean-Jacques Bertrand, chairman and CEO of Pasteur Mérieux Connaught; and Daniel Hoffmann, acting secretary of health for Pennsylvania.

They stood where Building 50 would rise, a structure that will house 446 people, including the departments of Clinical Research, Medical Affairs, Regulatory Affairs, Customer Account Management, and others. Some 230 people occupying temporary office space in more than 20 trailers will move into that building, which should be ready for occupancy by early 1998.

Before the groundbreaking, Williams thanked employees for their patience during the long wait for construction to begin. He especially thanked those who work in the trailers, many of whom may not know that Williams started his career at Connaught in a similar unit nearly 20 years earlier.

Bertrand told the crowd that as a group of companies, Pasteur Mérieux

Above: Breaking ground for Bldg. 50 in October 1996 are, from left: Georges Hibon, Jean-Jacques Bertrand, and Dave Williams.

Right: Georges Hibon speaks at groundbreaking ceremonies.

Facing page: Jean-Jacques Bertrand, architect of Vision 2000, addresses the crowd at groundbreaking.

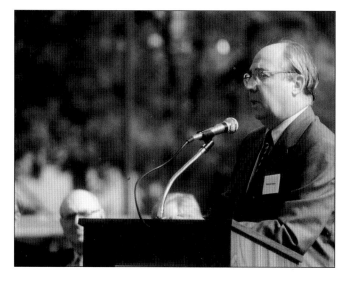

100

Connaught faces many challenges, including an increase in traditional diseases like meningitis, which will tax manufacturing capacity, and an increase in diseases like HIV (human immunodeficiency virus), tuberculosis, and pneumonia, which require an increased commitment to research. Swiftwater will play a key role in solving those challenges. "The construction of this building is a way of recognizing the importance of Swiftwater in the group."

After the luncheon, in the shade of a pine tree on the lawn of Building 45, Bertrand talked privately about the future of the Swiftwater site. As the architect of the group's Vision 2000 strategy, Bertrand has worked to support growth at Swiftwater, making investments in facilities that range from new equipment and other resources to the new addition to Building 45.

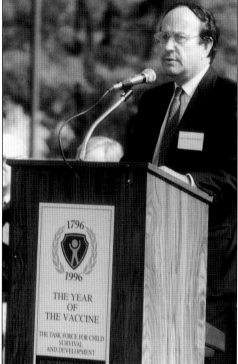

Developed under his tenure, the Pasteur Mérieux Connaught vision statement says it is the purpose of the company to "contribute, as a global leader, to the protection and maintenance of human health by creating superior immunological products for the prevention and treatment of infectious diseases and cancers." Vision 2000 defines the issues that are critical to the company: how it views itself, how it is viewed by stakeholders, and where it is heading. Vision 2000 provides general guidance and direction for all employees.

Swiftwater, Bertrand said, will play a major role in implementing that vision. "Research and Development will be stronger than it is today," he said. "We will have promising work here with major conjugate projects. Everything will be driven by innovation — new products, new vaccines. If we are successful in all of the projects we have, we will be a very prominent company in the global market. Swiftwater will be manufacturing products for the whole world."

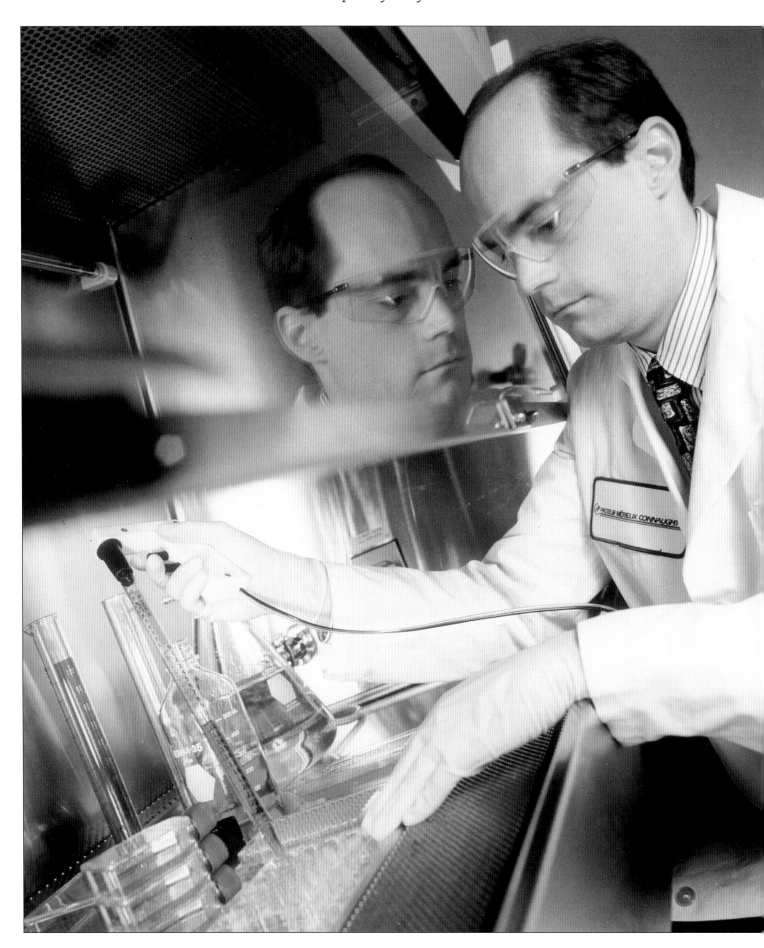

Going Global

Our people get the job done, even when they're given impossible odds. That's a tradition here.

— Phil Hosbach, director of Clinical Operations
and project leader for Tripedia® and TriHIBit™

Betting the Farm

*T*he stakes were enormous. Early in 1989, Dr. Howard Six walked into the office of Dave Williams with the proverbial good-news, bad-news scenario. The lawsuits and press coverage from the DTP scare had nearly ruined the company, along with most of the vaccine industry. Both knew the only way to survive was to produce a better diphtheria–tetanus–pertussis vaccine. The antigen of choice — an acellular pertussis component — was available in Japan. The good news was that Swiftwater had acquired this component from Biken and had gone into clinical trials, and the trials were going well.

As the first signs of green spread among the stone buildings of campus, Six, the vice president of Research and Development, delivered the bad news to his president: Through another Japanese company, Lederle Laboratories had done the same, and it looked as if Lederle would deliver its product first. Both men knew the first company to reach the market with what was perceived as a safer product would enjoy the accolades, as well as the profits.

The stakes were even higher for Swiftwater. The new technology embodied in the acellular vaccine would drive the industry into the next century, leading to the creation of an innovative pipeline and helping Swiftwater to differentiate its products from the competition. And finally, Swiftwater did not have the luxury of funding research and development with revenue from pharmaceutical sales. If Connaught Laboratories was ever going to be a world leader in pediatric vaccines, the company had to move quickly. That meant money. And that raised a concern. Swiftwater was no longer a single company; it was now part of Connaught Laboratories Ltd.

Facing page: The future dawns for Swiftwater with an influx of new talent and technology. Here, Gary Nabors conducts an experiment under an exhaust hood.

103

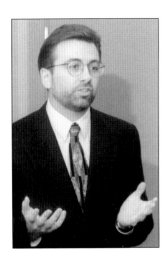

In Canada, Dr. Don Metzgar, senior vice president of Connaught Laboratories Ltd. and the person with the purse strings, listened to the story on the speakerphone. Dr. Six had a plan. Biken's clinical trials in Sweden had gone well. Under normal circumstances, Swiftwater would proceed step-by-step, waiting for each phase to be completed, analyzing the results, and then planning the next phase. But the labs did not have the time to proceed in sequence, not if it wanted to beat Lederle.

Swiftwater would plan the clinical trial phases in their entirety.

"Let's assume everything will work and do it all at one time," Six proposed.

Williams said he agreed. So did Metzgar. "If we're going to go for it, let's do it right," Metzgar said. "Let's increase the trials from 500 to 1,000. We'll double the budget."

"What about Lederle?" Six asked.

"We can catch them," Metzgar replied.

And they did. Through hard work, long hours, and innovative clinical-trial planning, Swiftwater became the first company to receive an FDA license for an acellular pertussis product for infants in the United States.

It was another example of a gutsy decision by Dave Williams and his team.

"This was the only hope we had to be first to market," he said. "Pertussis is an important product in pediatric immunization. It's often called the keystone of the pediatric vaccine marketplace. It was also the key in the coming combination vaccine market. The decision had more to do with strategic positioning in the marketplace."

Williams said the decision "would be challenged many times along the way" by people inside and outside the company.

Metzgar, too, was aware of the magnitude of the risk. "I authorized the doubling of the budget, the spending of 1.2 million in Canadian dollars," he said. "I had the authority to do so on paper, but I didn't have the funds."

The persistence showed by management paid well. After the U.S. Food and Drug Administration licensed booster doses of Tripedia in 1992, it licensed the vaccine for infants in 1996.

That strategy also allowed Swiftwater to capture a greater portion of the world biologicals market. Between 1985 and 1994, the U.S. vaccine market grew at a compounded annual rate of approximately 11%. During the same period, Swiftwater's revenue grew approximately 23%. Over the last decade, Swiftwater has seen tremendous progress. During that period, revenue grew from U.S. $30 million in 1985 to approximately U.S. $242 million in 1996.

Between 1997 and 2006, the U.S. vaccine market is expected to grow at a

Above: Phil Hosbach explains the theory behind Tripedia® at a news conference in Swiftwater.

Facing page: Damian Braga, vice president of Finance and Administration, and Dr. Howard Six, vice president of Research and Development, discuss strategy in 1997.

compound annual rate of about 14%, from slightly above U.S. $1 billion to more than U.S. $4 billion. Pasteur Mérieux Connaught anticipates its share of that market will grow from about 21% to about 33%, with most of the growth occurring in the pediatric, adolescent, and adult segments.

That kind of progress is sustained by innovation — in research and development, in marketing, in managing the resources the company possesses. As Swiftwater moves into the next century, it plans to broaden its product line, influence public policy on age-appropriate immunizations, and better manage the process of FDA approval. But as the gamble with Tripedia illustrates, the name of the game is research.

The Preeminence of R&D

In the 1990s, the Swiftwater Labs looked at the market's new emphasis on cost-cutting and decided that if it wanted to change managed care's perception of vaccines, it had to alter its own views on the subject.

"We shifted from selling undifferentiated commodities to marketing vital technology," said Damian Braga, vice president of Finance and Administration and one of the persons who develops Swiftwater's strategic plans. "We changed how we would view our products, from commodities to vaccines that are an essential part of health care. We started to place an emphasis on developing innovative products and being the first to market with them."

New Technologies

Senior management has learned well from the success of ProHIBiT and Tripedia. They have followed the example of Dr. Slee when he adapted the Pasteur Institute formula for the new technology of the time — glycerinated smallpox vaccine — and built a business from it. They understand the importance of innovation. Now, they intend to take science to the next level.

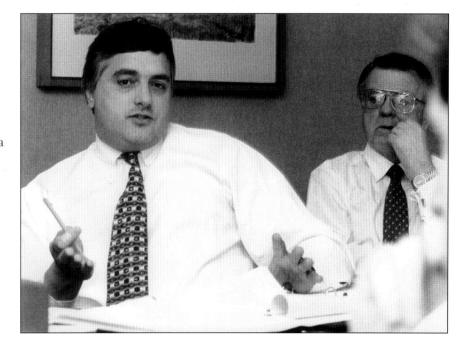

Conjugate and Recombinant Vaccines

Conjugates may hold the key to future vaccines for AIDS (acquired immunodeficiency syndrome), cancer, and even allergies. As Swiftwater prepares to enter the twenty-first century, it does so with a full pipeline of products that use that technology. Conjugate vaccines like ProHIBiT use a fragment, called a hapten, of a disease organism attached to a carrier protein molecule to induce immunity. Building on its own groundbreaking science, Swiftwater has launched a program to develop a pneumococcal polysaccharide conjugate vaccine intended for use in infants. The vaccine may also prevent an infection that plagues almost every child and parent, otitis media.

"As any parent knows, otitis media is a frustrating problem in young children, who always seem to come down with earaches," said Howard Six. "About 45% to 50% of otitis media is caused by *Streptococcus pneumoniae* organisms."

Pasteur Mérieux Connaught is also working on a vaccine for hepatitis A. Currently there are two licensed vaccines, one from Merck, the other from SmithKline. "Hepatitis A is a disease that occurs in adolescents but is widely spread," Six said. "We believe the vaccine will be used universally. It will fit into our emphasis on pediatric vaccines."

Manufactured by Pasteur Mérieux Connaught France, the vaccine has been licensed for use in that country and the U.K. Swiftwater started clinical trials in the United States in 1997 and is about 2 or 3 years away from FDA licensure.

Below: Pat Braun works on a conjugate project.

Facing page: The latest developments in technology are implemented in Manufacturing.

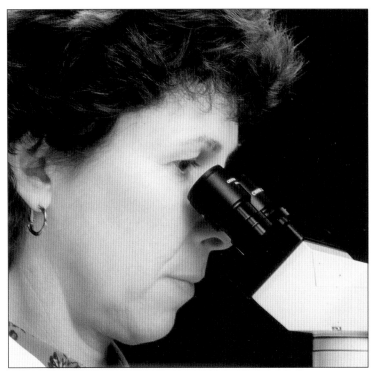

Viral Vectors

Swiftwater is also exploring the area of vector vaccines, an agent that transfers genetic material to the vaccinee. Vector technology uses, among other things, poxvirus and canary pox, an avian poxvirus that will not replicate in human cells. When the virus enters a cell, it produces proteins and induces the immune response; an infectious virus is not assembled.

"The immune response to antigens depends on how the body first encounters them," Dr. Six said. "How you present the antigen determines the response you get to it. The advantages of vectors are several-fold.

If you put the gene that encodes for the antigen for which you want an immune response in a vector, you can induce an optimal immune response. That would be much more efficient than giving a purified protein.

"Another advantage is that you will be able to give multiple proteins at the same time. In clinical trials, we have inserted the genes for seven proteins and generated immune response to all of them. This means you can make combination vaccines that will be carried by only one vector." And that means greater protection with fewer injections.

Recombinant Technology

Swiftwater is now working with recombinant DNA-derived proteins to produce vaccines of greater purity and effectiveness. Genetically engineered DNA (deoxyribonucleic acid) is prepared by transplanting or splicing genes from one species into the cells of a host organism of a different species. Such DNA becomes part of the host's genetic makeup and is replicated.

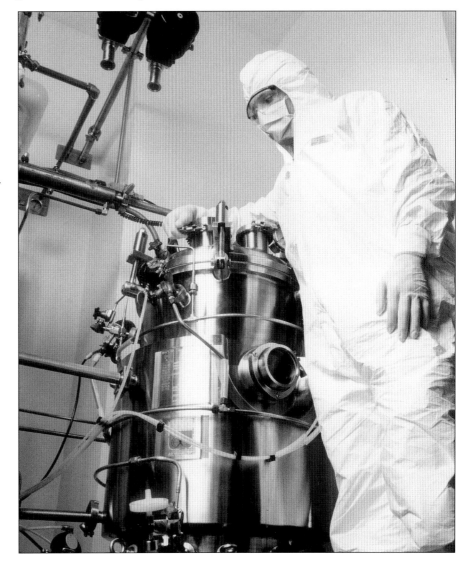

Swiftwater's R&D department is inserting genes into bacteria, yeast, and insect cells so that they will produce an antigen. The results are higher yields and easier purification. A practical application involves Lyme disease.

"Lyme borrelia is a difficult organism to grow," Six said. "It is expensive to grow and isolate the antigens from the organism. The ability to transfer genes into a system where the protein antigen is produced in large amounts makes it economical. What you're doing is fermentation, as in beer-making, only we use *Escherichia coli* instead of

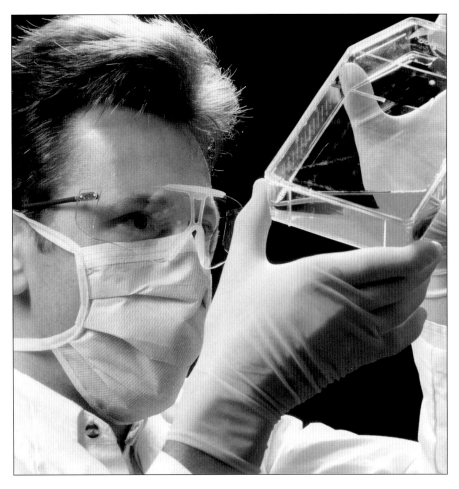

yeast, and it is modified to make the protein."

The ramifications for manufacturing are enormous, he said. "You can produce a much higher percentage of what you want."

DNA vaccines

For years, scientists believed foreign DNA in animals was nonfunctional — that is, there was no way to place DNA into a cell, or have it expressed, unless it was carried by a virus. Then researchers unexpectedly learned that certain forms of DNA, when injected, were taken up by the cells.

Swiftwater is investigating DNA technology because it could produce immune responses that persist for long periods of time. The labs are also addressing the safety concerns that arise from the new technology.

Other Vaccines

Also in the pipeline is a vaccine for zoster, also called shingles. The herpes zoster vaccine is used to prevent chicken pox, also called varicella. A second form of the disease causes shingles in adults.

"Currently there is one license for varicella, and that belongs to Merck," Six said. "We have developed a varicella vaccine in France. It is licensed for special use but not in the general population. It's anticipated we will develop the rest of the data in the United States and France."

Improving Existing Technologies

While Swiftwater has proven it can generate new products, it remains committed to improving existing ones. A case in point is its influenza vaccine.

Above: Don Walakomski of Research & Development conducts an experiment.

Facing page: Computers play an increasingly important role in R&D and production.

108

The Return of Flu

Influenza vaccines in general have been criticized over the years because their efficacy depends on how well they match the strains that are circulating among humans. The virus has the ability to change its antigenic character as it circulates throughout the population, and the Centers for Disease Control and Prevention, which provides the seed virus to manufacturers each year, has been hard-pressed to keep up.

While Fluzone met with great success in 1996 — Swiftwater manufactured about 40% of the influenza vaccine distributed in the United States — and its efficacy is well within the range of similar products (50% to 80%), Six said Swiftwater is working to further improve the vaccine.

Combination Vaccines

Ironically, the success of pediatric vaccines has created a new problem, one that is more social than medical. With so many infant diseases now preventable through vaccination, doctors and nurses are becoming concerned about the number of times they need to inoculate children during each visit to the office.

"To become fully immunized, a child can now receive three or four immunizations during a visit to the doctor," Six said. "Our goal is that, by the year

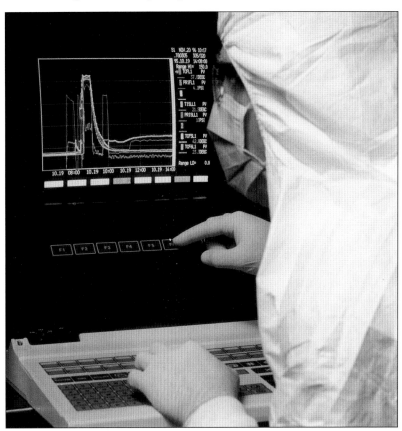

2000, we will have a vaccine that is a half-milliliter liquid product, so the child is fully immunized but only receives one inoculation for every visit to the doctor."

Swiftwater is making that transition in stages. Starting with Tripedia, the company has added a Hib conjugate to the product (TriHIBit™). "Then we'll skip to vaccines with six components: those four, a hepatitis B component, and the inactivated polio virus vaccine, IPOL®," the company's inactivated polio vaccine (IPV).

The strategy, Six said, "will increase our attractiveness to the public. It will show we have taken pains to put together all the antigens needed for these combination vaccines. We do not manufacture all of them, so we created partnerships to deliver the best product to our customers."

That foresight will also increase the quality of life for millions of children. "We have devoted considerable resources over the past 15 years to develop the best acellular pertussis vaccine we could. With IPV, we have committed time and resources to make a better and safer vaccine. These are issues of safety that go well beyond the convenience of patients."

Becoming part of a global organization also means combining vaccines from all over the world. Until 1992, Swiftwater produced and assembled all the components of DTP, which immunized against three diseases. After that year, it substituted the acellular pertussis component acquired from Biken in Japan to produce Tripedia, known generically as DTaP. The next combination vaccine matches Tripedia with ActHIB, a *Haemophilus influenzae* type b vaccine from France. That combination was licensed in late 1996 for the fourth, or booster, dose in children under the trade name TriHIBit and is expected to be licensed for infants in 1997. After that will come PRI, which will combine PedvaxHIB® *Haemophilus* b and Recombivax® HB from Merck with IPOL injectable inactivated polio vaccine from France. Shortly thereafter, Pasteur Mérieux Connaught, in partnership with Merck, plans to market ARBI, which will include ActHIB, Recombivax HB, Swiftwater's Tripedia (with its Biken component), and IPOL.

Total Submission Management

Outside the laboratory, Research and Development is speeding time to market by pioneering a process to reduce the time required to license a product. As part of a program called Total Submission Management, Swiftwater has partnered with the FDA in a pilot program to computerize data from clinical trials. In the past, Swiftwater has delivered up to 15 cartons of materials to the FDA. In the future, it plans to submit the license application electronically and put all clinical trial data on a CD-ROM disk for easier sorting.

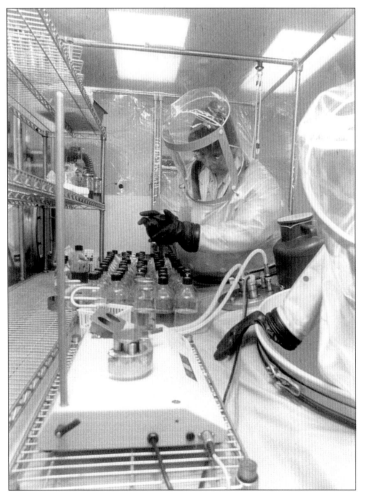

Below: Celeste Gesky and Dorothy Thorpe from the Sterility department use a barrier system to eliminate false positive readings.

"The database from a clinical trial is huge," Dr. Six said. "We analyze that data and send it to the FDA so they can see how we've done the analysis. We include all tests and analyses we've done. We believe this will speed both the submission process and the review process, because the FDA will have all of the information at its fingertips."

Partners in Profit

The relationship with other PMC group members in France and Canada will give Swiftwater the edge in dealing with changing technologies and markets throughout the world. Dave Williams said that cohesiveness benefits all members of the group:

> Being part of Pasteur Mérieux Connaught gives us the largest critical mass for developing and marketing products throughout the world. From a research, development, and manufacturing perspective, we're part of a global company that has the best capacity to get products ready for the market, and we play a role in that development and manufacturing. We benefit from what happens in Canada and France, and vice versa. From a marketing perspective, we can draw on products manufactured throughout the world by Pasteur Mérieux Connaught. That will allow us to have an excellent pipeline and a steady supply of product that will be second-to-none over time.

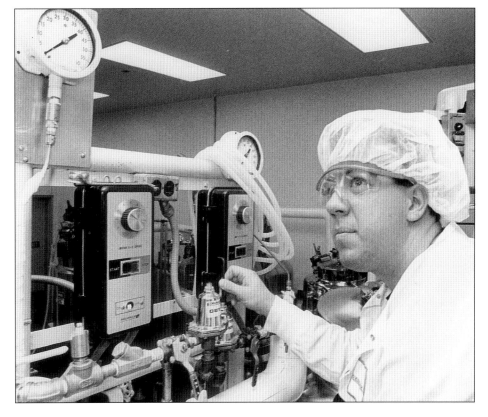

Below: Mike Stirr in the 'penthouse' of the influenza manufacturing facility, concentrating the virus.

Partnerships with other companies will also be crucial, he added. "We have to be able to identify emerging technologies, seek them out, and enter into joint ventures if we're going to be effective in competing against a company such as Lederle or SmithKline."

What makes that work, and what makes Swiftwater an attractive partner, is its track record. "We have demonstrated that we can successfully develop, manufacture, and commercialize vaccines and other biological products," he said. "That's a significant advantage."

Below: Derek Pyle, research technician in Molecular Biology, pours gel for a DNA sequencing test.

Facing page: A dedicated worker trundles eggs into the incubator during the height of flu-production season.

Building the Future

In 1892, Dr. Richard Slee became infected with cholera and retreated to the mountains of Pennsylvania to recuperate. Eighty years later, National Drug began marketing a vaccine to prevent the disease, an acute infection of the small intestine that causes severe dehydration and depletion of electrolytes. In the intervening years, world health officials thought they had virtually eliminated cholera from the globe. But between 1991 and 1993, more than 90,000 cases were reported in Central and South America alone.

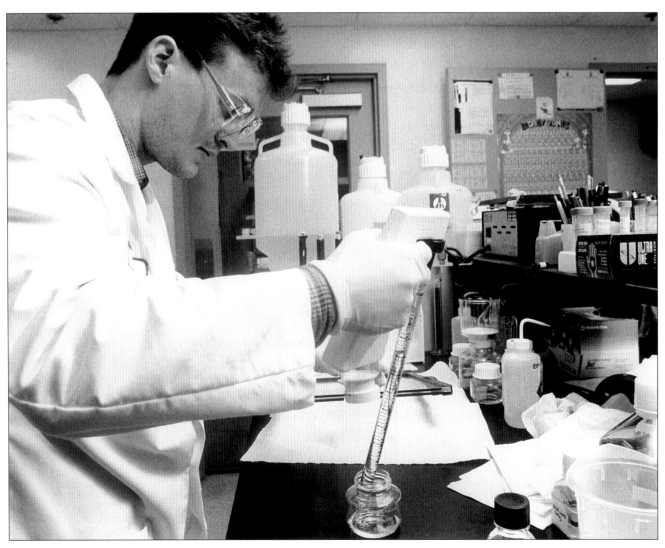

Cholera is not the only infectious disease to make a comeback. Microbes that cause strep throat, pneumonia, tuberculosis, rheumatic fever, meningitis, osteomyelitis, and salmonella are showing an increasing resistance to antibiotics. Even the bubonic plague has revisited itself on India.

Throughout the Pasteur Mérieux Connaught organization, the global spread of preventable diseases has raised a call to arms. Over the past century, the Swiftwater Labs have moved from stone buildings and stables to multi-million-dollar manufacturing facilities capable of supplying the market in Canada and the United States. In recent years, administrative and support facilities have also been built to provide workspace for the significant increase in employees at the site. As world demand for its products grows, the once retiring laboratories in the woods of Pennsylvania now stand center stage in a race to control a global resurgence of disease.

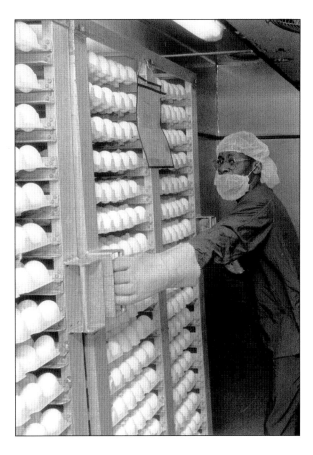

Transfer of Technology

In 1996, the Pasteur Mérieux Connaught marketing forecast showed the world-wide demand for vaccines would increase beyond the groups' capacity to meet that need. In response, the organization reevaluated its global manufacturing facilities and capacities to determine the fastest and best approach to meet that challenge. Sites were identified where products could be logically transferred. The transfer was necessary for three reasons: to take advantage of existing capacity; to get maximum use from existing facilities; and to eliminate duplication wherever possible, such as manufacturing the same vaccine at multiple sites.

In the future, the products that will be manufactured in Swiftwater include meningococcal polysaccharide, meningococcal conjugate, and pneumococcal conjugate vaccines. Swiftwater will manufacture influenza vaccine for the world market until it reaches its capacity. At that point, further market demands would be supplied from the French sites.

Other planned product transfers include polio and rabies vaccines from Canada to France and hepatitis A vaccine from France to Canada. Canada has been named the global manufacturing site for diphtheria and tetanus vaccines.

In addition to product transfer, technology transfer has been a conduit for process, and ultimately product, improvement. One example of this exchange involves influenza vaccine production. Through the sharing of technology, a chemical-splitting process used in the United States was incorporated in the French process, resulting in higher yields and reduced manufacturing costs. At the same time, an innovative egg harvester designed in France was incorporated in the U.S. influenza vaccine manufacturing process. The French design has advantages over the traditional harvester, allowing for increased viral recovery from the egg and ultimately higher yields and lower costs.

Gary Ebbert, vice president of Operations in Swiftwater, described the process of collaboration:

> We will use Pasteur Mérieux Connaught's core competencies to become a global supplier in the areas where we are the experts.

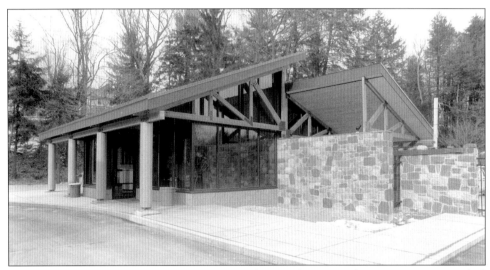

Influenza production will continue to be one area where we have a technological advantage. Meninge, pneumo, and Lyme vaccines are other products that we will manufacturer because of our experience with fermentation, polysaccharide purification, and conjugation. We are becoming a global partner, leveraging the things we do best.

That strategy "inspires us to focus on innovative technology to develop vaccines for the entire world," Ebbert said. "Cost becomes a significant competitive issue in manufacturing. We need to be creative in order to be the low-cost producer."

Above: The new reception center replaced the guardhouse in May 1997.

Facing page: Dave Williams, right, with Monte Kramer, vice president of Human Resources, in 1997.

The Capital Program

To prepare for the transfers, Swiftwater has developed an approximately $60 million capital plan from 1997 to 2000. In addition to the administration center construction, the program calls for a scale-up for pneumo polysaccharide, pneumo conjugate, and meninge conjugate manufacturing. Swiftwater plans to upgrade Research and Development buildings, replace equipment, and retrofit heating and electrical systems. In Quality Control and Quality Assurance, the laboratories will continue their initiatives in document imaging, global laboratory information management systems, and laboratory testing.

In the long run, Swiftwater plans to restructure Manufacturing to shorten product-cycle times, expand distribution facilities, and construct a new Quality Operations facility. In Marketing, the company will increase its focus on customer-oriented product presentations, such as detachable preprinted patient labels, bar coding, and electronic vaccine tracking.

Global Reach

Despite the fashionable saying that the world is shrinking, the people in Swiftwater have dealt with that reality for years. Driving the system through the 1980s was a vaccine technology that depended on inactivated bacterial toxins,

like tetanus, whole-cell killed bacteria, like pertussis, and attenuated live viruses, like oral polio. That scenario changed with the advent of Tripedia and TriHIBit, with sophisticated components and finished vaccines that are sourced and shipped throughout the world. One hundred years after the establishment of the Swiftwater Labs, the site that introduced the United States to a new French product has taken its place in the international arena.

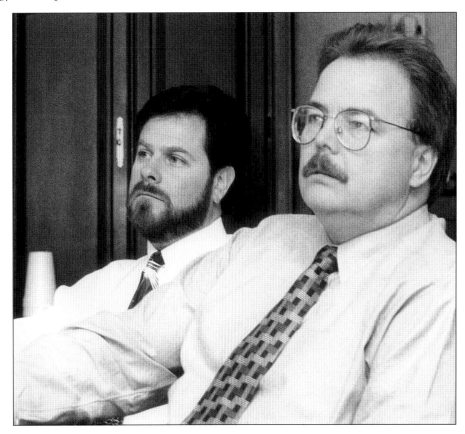

That means new products, new licensure requirements, and new technology to carry out that mission. To coordinate a project of this magnitude, Pasteur Mérieux Connaught will move to the next generation of its computer forecast system, called Enterprise Resource Planning, or ERP. The upgraded system will forecast global supply and demand and help Swiftwater and other partners allocate resources and generate schedules to meet that demand. The $15 million to $20 million investment will create a shared system throughout the Pasteur Mérieux Connaught group.

ERP is part of a technological strategy called IS 2000. "It is a new, integrated computer system that will replace several current systems as a tool for aiding Manufacturing, Distribution, Purchasing, and Finance," said Braga. "The first phase, completed in 1996, involved developing process coordination among sites for production, inventory management, and order fulfillment. Full implementation is expected by the end of 1998."

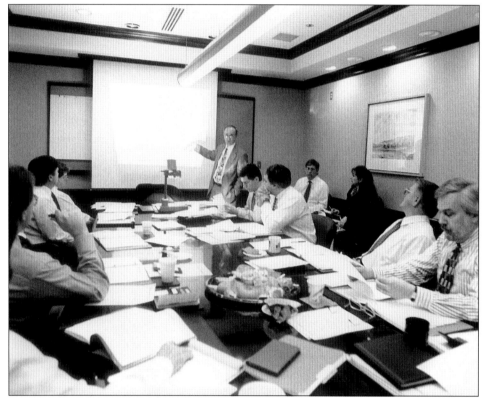

IS 2000 will allow the sharing of information among Pasteur Mérieux Connaught's four business units, four production sites, and four legal entities.

Sharing is key to success in global markets, and not just in the area of technology. In marketing, all members of Pasteur Mérieux Connaught are sharing best practices, exchanging information on what works. Yet each site retains its identity. "While we are trying to share success globally, the corporate strategy is to let each operating unit focus on the unique opportunities in its market," Braga said. "Swiftwater has a global responsibility on the manufacturing and supply side, but our sales and marketing efforts are focused on the U.S. market."

While he expects the global market will continue to become more competitive, he also believes the old adage that there is strength in numbers. "Swiftwater used to operate on its own. Now we are a major part of a global company."

The company has achieved that synthesis because its employees have embraced an entrepreneurial, can-do spirit for the past 100 years, whether alone or as part of a larger group.

"We've always been the small guy on the block," said Williams, "but we've always been resourceful and aggressive enough to seize an opportunity and

Above: Senior management reviews strategy in the executive conference room of Bldg. 45 in early 1997.

Facing page: Contractors pour the foundation for Bldg. 50, spring of 1997.

make something good happen. In this business, you have to focus on the things that make a difference. There is no other way to succeed. We are focused on vaccines, and what our resources will allow us to do. If you follow that approach, you can out-finesse and out-maneuver the competition."

Phil Hosbach, director of Clinical Operations and project leader for Tripedia and TriHIBit, characterized that resourcefulness another way. "Sometimes we don't have the appropriate resources, but the people here are so dedicated, they make things happen, sometimes through sheer dint of will. Even when they are given impossible odds, our people get the job done. That's a tradition here."

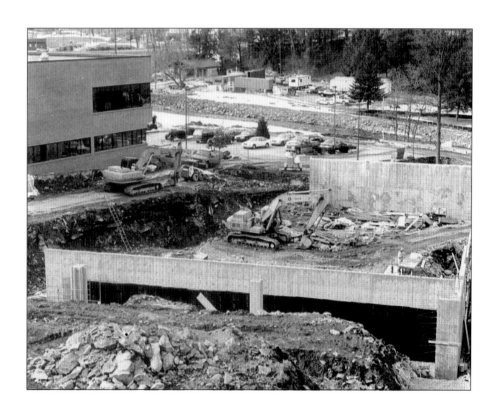

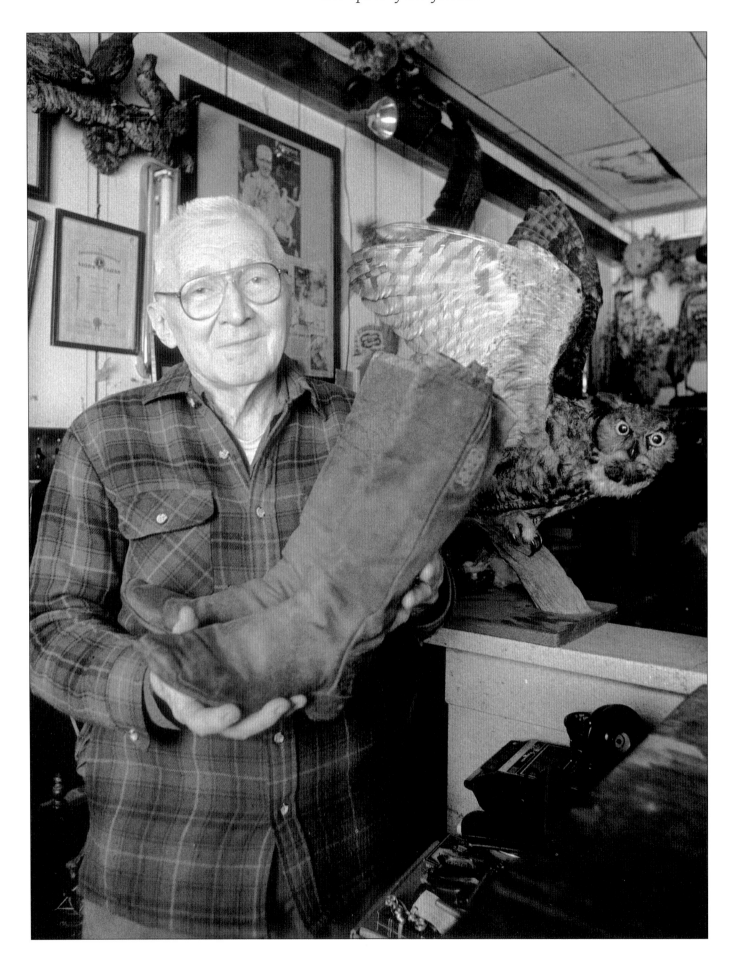

Epilogue

*A*s they walked to a conference room a few doors from the office of
Dave Williams, Willard Webster, Tony Bolyn, and Don Metzgar swapped war
stories about the old days — times when the three of them ran the Swiftwater
laboratories. While Metzgar visits the campus regularly as a consultant, Webster,
who lives in Gwynedd near Norristown, Pennsylvania, and Bolyn, who lives
within a few miles of the labs, had not seen the facilities in years. As they walked
toward the executive conference room of Building 45, they peeked into cubicles
and smiled in amazement at the staff, the paperwork, and the machinery.

"I'm very impressed," Bolyn said. "The growth is remarkable. Compared with
the growth of years ago, the development in recent times is amazing.
Everywhere you look, you see growth. I remember when we had a total
employee population of less than a dozen. Today it's a thousand or more. The
physical facilities we had just can't compare with today."

Bolyn was also impressed with the company's standing in the community, as
it makes the transition from a modest curiosity to major employer. "The company at Swiftwater has become a very respectable institution," he said. "The people
are viewed as scientists of the first order."

Webster agreed with Bolyn's comments on growth. "I am amazed," he said,
looking around the facility. "Certainly when Connaught took over, I don't think
gross sales were more than 2 million or 3 million dollars a year."

In his office down the hall, Dave Williams nursed a coffee in a Styrofoam cup
and thought about the future.

"Where will we be in 10 years?" he asked, raising his eyebrows. "By the year
2010, I would hope all of the products we have in the pipeline would be in the
marketplace. In my wildest dreams, for the needs of this country, I hope that
someone has solved the HIV dilemma. And I would see a strong, viable company that has the broadest line of vaccines in the United States, one that is part of
Pasteur Mérieux Connaught. We have 1,100 employees today; I wouldn't be
surprised if we have double that by the year 2010."

He glanced out the window at a parking lot filled with cars, a new bridge
over the Swiftwater Creek, Metzgar's Pond swimming with ducks. "I see nothing but good things ahead."

Facing page:
Surrounded by
memorabilia from
47 years of work
at the Swiftwater
Labs, Clair
Wallingford holds
a pair of boots
that once
belonged to
Arthur Slee.
Wallingford's
store/museum is
in Appenzell,
Pennsylvania.

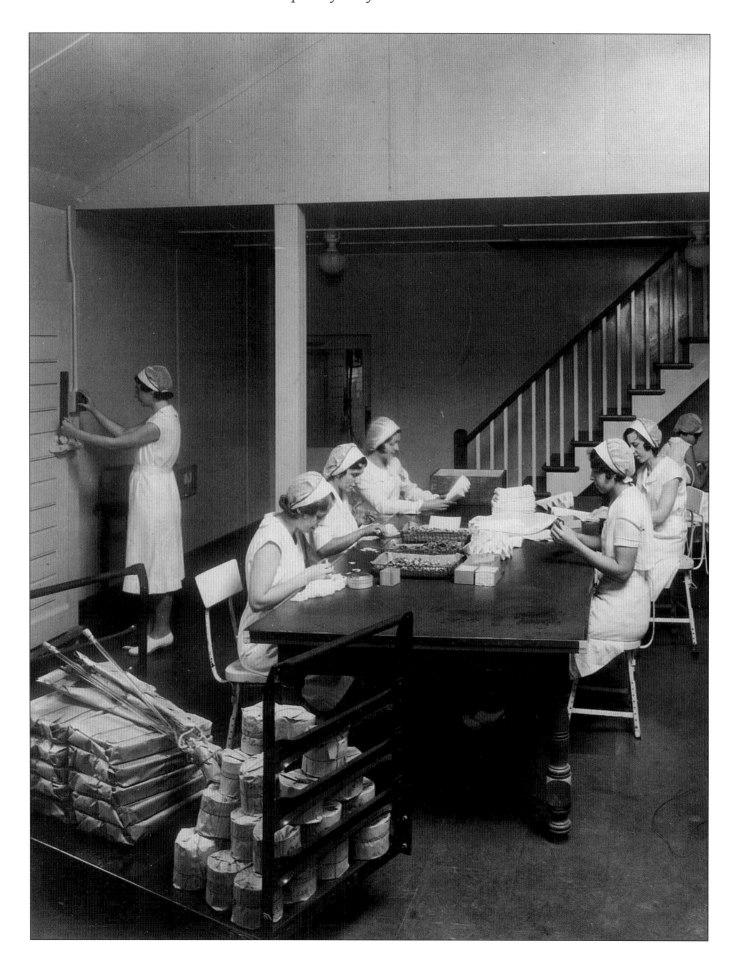

Appendixes

Appendix A

Historical figures of the Swiftwater Laboratories

Bolyn, Dr. Anthony E. Joined the Biological Laboratories in 1938 upon his graduation from Lehigh University and left the following year to pursue his studies at Purdue University. After graduating from Purdue, he returned to the laboratories in 1943, completing work to earn his doctorate. In the early 1960s, he worked as associate director of the Biological Laboratories at Swiftwater, responsible for Manufacturing and Development. His job was to coordinate the preparation of National's serums and vaccines, as well as improve manufacturing procedures and the quality of products. He played a role in National's 1957 response to the Asian flu crisis. In July 1985, Connaught Laboratories Inc. dedicated Building 32, Quality Control, in his name. He retired in 1980.

Carr, Charles E. Former chairman of the board of National Drug and founder of the Twenty Year Club, organized on March 20, 1945, to honor employees with at least 20 years of service. Building 4 is named after him. In 1900, Carr joined National Drug in New York. With G. F. Harvey, its first president, and Leon Harvey, he formed the first board of directors. A year later, Carr was elected to the office of treasurer. In 1906, National moved its headquarters from New York to Philadelphia. Carr was elected president in 1928, two years before National purchased the Swiftwater Labs. In 1943, he was elected chairman of the board, succeeded as president by Alfred B. Collins. Subsequent National presidents include H. R. Marschalk, Charles M. McCallister, and Jim Dodd.

Davies, Alun. President of Connaught Laboratories Ltd. of Canada and Connaught Laboratories Inc. in America during and after the acquisition in 1978. Originally from the United Kingdom, he worked with the Wellcome Foundation before arriving in Toronto. Helped negotiate the agreement with the Salk Institute.

Facing page: Finishing room at National Drug, Swiftwater, circa 1932.

Diefenderfer, Barbara Edwards Slee. Second wife of Arthur Slee. Daughter of a prominent Stroudsburg attorney. Now living near Lebanon, Pennsylvania.

Fisher, Dorothy Canfield. Novelist and wife of John Redwood Fisher, son of Dr. William R. Fisher. Died November 9, 1958, in Vermont at the age of 79. Her books include *Vermont Tradition: The Biography of an Outlook*, published in 1953.

Fisher, Dr. William Redwood. Partner with Dr. Richard Slee in the Pocono Biological Laboratories from 1901–08. Married Elisabeth Virginia Jennings. Had four children: William Redwood Fisher Jr., who died in infancy; Elizabeth Lewis, who did not marry; Ester Lewis, who did not marry; and John Redwood Fisher, who married the writer Dorothy Canfield. Born in Mobile, Ala., November 1, 1844. His father, Samuel S. Fisher, died in 1848 of yellow fever. Settled in Hoboken in 1874. Moved to Swiftwater in 1901 and built a brownstone at the junction of Routes 611 and 314 that now houses Kelly Antiques. During World War I, the Fishers lived in France for 3 years while he served in the American Ambulance Field Service. He died on March 28, 1926, at his home in Swiftwater.

Knerr, Russell P. Joined National Drug in 1927 and spent a year in the laboratories at 5109 Germantown Avenue. When National acquired the Slee Laboratories, he was sent to Swiftwater to take charge of sterility testing and the production of toxins. Knerr functioned in every capacity, even injecting and bleeding horses. In 1942, he was appointed director of the laboratories, taking the place of Arthur Slee, who was promoted to director of the biological division of National Drug. He retired in 1962.

Maginnis, Arthur. Husband of Ella Maginnis, father of Ella Maginnis Slee. Died July 10, 1891. Ran the Swiftwater Inn, on the western side of Route 611, for more than 20 years. His property on the eastern side of Route 611 became Slee's in 1897.

Maginnis, Ella. Wife of Arthur Maginnis. Mother of Ella, who married Dr. Richard M. Slee. Died November 21, 1913, in Swiftwater.

Metzgar, Dr. Don P. Began work at Swiftwater, then National Drug, in 1966 as senior virologist. Was the director of Biological Research and Manufacturing in Swiftwater in the mid–1970s. In 1978, he was appointed vice president of Operations in Swiftwater. From 1982 to 1984 he worked as vice president of Operations for CLL in Canada. He returned from CLL in July 1984 as vice president of Operations at Swiftwater. In April 1988, he once again moved to Toronto, when he was named senior vice president of CLL, retiring in 1994.

Palmer, A. Mitchell. Attorney for Richard Slee. Palmer is the only person from Monroe County to attain cabinet rank. He served as U.S. attorney general under Woodrow Wilson. He is known for rounding up aliens during the Red Scare of 1920.

Regan, Ellen. Second secretary at National Drug's Swiftwater laboratories, replacing Merlin Rutt, who assumed other duties. Joined in 1942 as a finisher; retired in 1989 with 47 years of service. Worked for Russell Knerr, the director, until he retired, then for Dr. Anthony Bolyn.

Salk, Dr. Jonas Edward. Microbiologist. Born 1914; died 1995. Developed the first vaccine effective against poliomyelitis in 1952. After massive field tests in 1953 and 1954, the vaccine quickly came into wide use in 1955 and helped to reduce the incidence of polio until an oral vaccine was introduced by Albert Bruce Sabin in 1960.

Slee, Arthur Maginnis. Son of Ella Maginnis Slee and Richard M. Slee. Born in Swiftwater on May 6, 1894. Died in Stroudsburg on December 11, 1968, at the age of 74. He joined the company as a partner in 1911, when his father returned from New York to reopen the laboratories. Took over for his father during World War I. He received his basic training at the Medical School of New York University and in the research laboratories of the New York City Department of Health. Served as captain, Sanitary Corps, U.S. Army, during World War I. When the labs were leased by National Drug in 1927, he was retained as director, serving until 1937, when he assumed additional duties as associate director of the Biological Division of National. In 1941 he relinquished active supervision of the lab and established headquarters at the main offices of the company in Philadelphia as director of the Biological Division. He retired in 1945.

Slee, Ella Maginnis. Born on August 30, 1870, the daughter of Arthur and Ella Maginnis of Swiftwater. Died in East Stroudsburg on September 1, 1943, at the age of 73. Wife of Dr. Richard Slee, whom she married on November 1, 1892, in Swiftwater.

Slee, Phoebe Edmunds. First wife of Arthur Slee. Born November 23, 1892, in Lynchburg, Virginia. Died March 13, 1964, in Stroudsburg at the age of 78. She was the daughter of James Easley and Harriet Prescott Edmunds. They had one son, Richard E. Slee, and two grandchildren, Prescott W. Slee and Deborah W. Slee. She attended Randolph Macon Women's College in Lynchburg.

Slee, Richard Child. Father of founder Dr. Richard Slee. Husband of Maria J. (Orr) Slee. Died in Swiftwater on May 1, 1912, at the age of 69. A native of Canada, he and his wife settled in Brooklyn, N.Y., where he engaged in a dry goods business. After retiring, active in the Swiftwater Methodist church.

Slee, Richard M. (Dr., Col.). Founder of Pocono Biological Laboratories. Born September 15, 1867, in Brooklyn, N.Y.; died April 8, 1945, in Stroudsburg. Founded the laboratories in 1897. Closed them in 1908; reopened the facility in 1911. In 1923, he joined the staff of the New York State Department of Health, serving later as deputy commissioner of health in West Chester County, N.Y. Sold the Slee Laboratories to the National Drug Co. in 1930. Retired from West Chester on October 1, 1937. Lived his last 2 years in Stroudsburg. He wrote one novel, with Cornelia A. Pratt, entitled *Dr. Berkeley's Discovery*, about a pathologist who solves a murder by "developing" brain tissue much like a photographer processes film. It was published by G. P. Putnam's Sons, New York, in 1899.

Sorrentino, Dr. James. After working at Walter Reed Army Institute of Research, he joined the staff in Swiftwater in August 1967. Largely responsible for the development of Fluzone® and Menomune®, and bringing the K-2 centrifuge to Swiftwater. Promoted to director of Manufacturing and Development in the early 1970s. In 1974, he accepted a job at Richardson–Merrell headquarters in Cincinnati, Ohio.

Wallingford, Clair. Born in 1919, he joined National Drug in 1938 as a laborer, washing bottles and tubes in the kitchen. Known for his collection of laboratory memorabilia at his store in Appenzell, Pennsylvania. Retired in December 1984.

Webster, G. Willard. Joined the Swiftwater Laboratories in 1950. Responsible for bringing production of yellow fever and epidemic typhus vaccines to the company. Also introduced the operation for freeze-drying. Mechanized the Filling and Labeling department. Helped design and construct virtually all of the company's manufacturing buildings. Dr. Jonas Salk paid special tribute to him in 1977 for his contributions to the vaccine industry. The pair worked together in the summer of 1942 in the preparation of the first batch of influenza virus vaccine ever field-tested. Promoted to the number-two spot with National Drug in 1960. Retired in 1978. Building 37, the influenza manufacturing facility, was named after him in February 1988.

Appendix B

Achievements of the Swiftwater Laboratories

Produced the first glycerinated smallpox vaccine in the United States in 1897. Reduced side effects from vaccination. Used by the U.S. Army to immunize all soldiers during the Spanish–American War.

Introduced the first purified tetanus toxoid vaccine developed and manufactured in the United States in 1933. Also produced the first purified diphtheria toxoid in the nation.

Produced the first commercially successful triple-immunization vaccine, diphtheria–tetanus–pertussis, or DTP, in April 1944.

Created the world's first zonally purified influenza vaccine, using the K-2 centrifuge developed by the Atomic Energy Commission at Oak Ridge, Tenn., for the enrichment of uranium. Other firsts associated with the process include: egg harvesters featuring a vacuum-assisted harvest needle; high-volume inoculators; control manifold for routing processed fluids featuring the first stainless-steel disconnects in the industry; egg decapitator knives; and devices that monitored and controlled the process.

Created the first commercial polysaccharide vaccine, Menomune®.

Created the world's first licensed conjugate vaccine. On December 22, 1987, ProHIBiT® became the first vaccine prepared through conjugate technology to be licensed by the FDA for use in humans. The *Haemophilus* b capsular polysaccharide is chemically linked to diphtheria toxoid. It is used for routine immunization of children against diseases caused by *Haemophilus influenzae* type b.

Became sole distributor of inactivated polio vaccine (IPV) in the United States. In 1987, the FDA approved a license for CLL to manufacture an inactivated polio vaccine, Poliovax®, followed by PMsv's IPOL®.

Became the sole U.S. manufacturer of yellow fever vaccine in 1952.

Became the first company in the United States to market a DTaP vaccine for infant indications. The vaccine, Tripedia®, combines an acellular pertussis component with diphtheria and tetanus toxoids to provide a safer product.

Appendix C

A Brief History of the Property at Swiftwater

1896. Dr. Richard M. Slee, a pathologist, establishes a laboratory, known as the Pocono Biological Laboratories, to produce glycerinated smallpox vaccine on the property of his in-laws at Swiftwater.

1897. The first building is completed and approved by the Pennsylvania State Board of Health. The first vaccine is sold.

1898. The laboratory supplies smallpox vaccine to the U.S. armed forces during the Spanish–American War.

1901. Dr. Slee and Dr. William R. Fisher, chief surgeon of Bellevue Hospital in New York, form a partnership to operate the laboratories.

1903. The U.S. Secretary of the Treasury issues licenses to biological manufacturers. The Pocono laboratories receive license number 6, for smallpox vaccine.

December 1908. The laboratories close and the partnership is dissolved. Slee moves to New York to become director of Lederle Antitoxin Laboratory.

1911. Slee returns to Swiftwater and reopens the laboratory under the name of the Slee Laboratories. Glycerinated smallpox vaccine and tetanus antitoxin are produced. Slee's son, Arthur, becomes a partner.

1927. Dr. H. K. Mulford, director of research for the National Drug Company of Philadelphia, leases the Slee Laboratories with the option to buy. There are nine employees.

1930. National Drug purchases the Slee Laboratories and continues biological production under license number 101. Richard Slee and his wife Ella sell approximately 47 acres to National on May 26.

February 27, 1956. The Vick Chemical Co. purchases National, which continues to operate as a wholly owned subsidiary.

December 1960. Vick Chemical changes its name to Richardson–Merrell Inc. National merges into RMI as an operating division.

September 27, 1963. J. Burton Hamblin and his wife sell 10 acres to National Drug.

November 17, 1970. A. Byrd and Mary McDowell sell 100.44 acres to National Drug.

September 1971. The National Drug Co. division consolidates with the Wm. S. Merrell division to form the Merrell–National Laboratories division of Richardson–Merrell Inc., which operates from Cincinnati.

December 31, 1977. Merrell–National Laboratories division of RMI withdraws from the biological vaccine business. The entire business — along with the land, buildings, equipment, supplies, and all other assets located at Swiftwater — are donated to the Salk Institute for Biological Studies, headquartered in La Jolla, Calif.

The Salk Institute sells the manufacturing facilities and equipment to Connaught Laboratories Inc., a subsidiary of Connaught Laboratories Ltd. of Toronto, Canada, and retains one building for military research.

January 1, 1978. CLI begins operations at Swiftwater.

December 13, 1989. The Canadian government allows the acquisition of Connaught BioSciences Inc. stock by Institut Mérieux of Lyon, France.

November 1, 1996. Connaught begins doing business under the name Pasteur Mérieux Connaught.

Appendix D

Chronology of Acquisitions

1896. Dr. Richard Slee establishes the Pocono Biological Laboratories in Swiftwater, Pennsylvania. Production begins the following year.

1908. Slee closes the Swiftwater lab and moves to New York State.

1911. Slee reopens the Swiftwater facility as the Slee Laboratories.

1927. The National Drug Co. leases the Swiftwater property. It exercises an option to buy in 1930.

1938. Vick Chemical Co. acquires one of the oldest pharmaceutical manufacturers in the United States, the Wm. S. Merrell Co.

1956. National Drug sold to Vick Corp. for $6.5 million.

1961. Richardson–Merrell Inc. (RMI) absorbs National Drug as a division.

1971. RMI begins consolidation of its two domestic ethical pharmaceutical divisions, National Drug and the Wm. S. Merrell Co., calling the company Merrell–National Laboratories.

1978. RMI donates the facility to the Salk Institute, a not-for-profit medical research organization based in California, originated by Dr. Jonas Salk, developer of the first polio vaccine. Salk sells the manufacturing portion to Connaught Laboratories Ltd. of Toronto and keeps the Army labs on the hill.

July 8, 1987. Institut Mérieux, a major vaccine producer 50.8% of which is owned by the Rhône–Poulenc Group, purchases a 12.6% stake in Canada Development Corp. (CDC) Life Sciences. That company controls Canada's major vaccines and blood derivatives producer, Connaught Laboratories Ltd., as well as Montreal BioResearch.

December 1989. Institut Mérieux S.A. buys 100 percent of Connaught BioSciences Inc. Based in Lyon, France, Institut Mérieux is a diversified biologics company with a human–health business accounting for 50% of its sales, with the balance composed of veterinary and other products. In 1988, revenues from its human–health business were $351.9 million.

April 1994. The Rhône–Poulenc Group acquires Pasteur Mérieux Connaught.

Appendix E

Construction Time Line

1897. Construction of the first structure, Building 3, holding offices and later manufacturing. Later used for Product Development.

1911. Building 6 constructed as a stable for nearly eight horses needed to produce tetanus toxoid. Building 8 erected to house the manufacturing for that product. Building 8 later became the Laundry and then the Centennial Conference Center, for the display of historical artifacts.

1913. Building 1 constructed as the home of Dr. Richard and Ella Slee, to replace "Ivy," the Slee's original home, which had burned prior to that. Later, Building 1 served as a dormitory for male employees, then housed Medical Affairs, Product Development, Research Administration, and Human Resources.

1931. Building 4, the Carr building, constructed for use as a laboratory.

1932. Building 11 finished. Originally located where Building 21 now stands, it was later moved, then demolished. Its second floor, an attic, was the site's first maintenance shop.

1939. Building 6C, an additional horse stable, built.

1940. Building 31, Quality Control animal quarters and storage, constructed. Buildings 11 and 12 are demolished.

1951. Building 6F, Biological Services and later called Building 7, finished. Addition made to back of Building 3. Building 13, the Quonset hut, added as a warehouse and refitted in 1981 as a research lab.

1952. Since production of yellow fever vaccine required an isolated facility, Building 14 constructed. First generation of freeze-drying equipment installed in Building 3. Building 15 demolished.

1958. Three buildings remodeled: Building 19, hazardous plant storage; Building 20, the boiler house; and Building 21, the pertussis laboratory. Building 21 was originally constructed as a lab for researching upper respiratory vaccines. Later, it was leased for a government R&D program and used as a National Drug warehouse.

1960. Addition of the 100,000-gallon water tower, Building 41.

1961. Construction started on Buildings 24 and 25.

1962. Building 28 erected as an animal test area for a government contract. By 1980 it was used for influenza manufacturing. Building 29, the sewage treatment plant and lagoons, and Building 36, the well pump pit, constructed. Building 30 removed.

1963. Buildings 24 and 25, the $2 million biological research complex, completed to house developmental work on a variety of vaccines for the army.

1964. To provide larger Quality Control and animal testing facilities, Building 32, later dedicated as the Bolyn Building, finished.

1965. Biological Services Storage, Building 33, built.

1966. Building 34, Alcohol Solvent Storage, completed. Building 35, the Pennsylvania Power & Light Co. power main, finished.

1971. Building 37, the Influenza Vaccine Production Building, a series of laboratories designed for the manufacture of National's zonal-purified influenza vaccine, built. It was later dedicated as the G. Willard Webster Building.

1971. Plans drafted for construction of the $355,000 Smallpox Production Facility.

1972. The Influenza Vaccine Production Facility, now a 26,500-square-foot facility, completed.

1978. Building 5 added for tetanus manufacturing.

1980. Building 38 added to Building 37 for warehouse and distribution activities. Cafeteria added to Building 21. The new sterile filling and packaging addition to Building 37 was nearly finished. Buildings 42, 43, and 44 removed.

1984. Building 27, the plant waste compactor/glass grinder, built.

1987. The CDC Life Sciences Inc. Board of Directors granted approval for the construction of a $10.8 million biological manufacturing building on the CLI campus. Guardhouse and Building 21 (pertussis manufacturing) completed.

1988. Building 45, the $4 million administrative support building, completed. Warehouse addition completed at Building 38.

1989. Building 46 (biological manufacturing) completed.

1996. Construction began on a $9 million addition to Building 45, the administration center, to be called Building 50.

1997. Building 8, constructed in 1911 as a tetanus facility and later used as the Laundry, was renovated to serve as the Centennial Conference Center and archive for the display of historical materials. Construction began on a bridge over the Swiftwater Creek and a 1,200-square-foot Reception Center that replaced the guardhouse at the main gate. Building 20 was expanded to house a third boiler to accommodate an increase in vaccine production.

Appendix F

Products of Pasteur Mérieux Connaught USA

ActHIB®. *Haemophilus* b conjugate vaccine (tetanus toxoid conjugate).

DT. Diphtheria and tetanus toxoids adsorbed, USP (for pediatric use).

DTP. Diphtheria and tetanus toxoids and pertussis vaccine, adsorbed, USP (for pediatric use).

Diphtheria Antitoxin USP. Used to counter the effects of toxins produced by the bacillus *Corynebacterium diphtheriae*, which cause difficulty in breathing, high fever, and weakness.

Fluzone®. Influenza virus vaccine, whole virion and subvirion. For the prevention of influenza in all age groups, especially those 65 and older and others with chronic debilitating conditions. Developed at Swiftwater in the late 1960s. Process was further refined through collaboration with the Atomic Energy Laboratories in Oak Ridge, Tenn., which had the only large-scale centrifuges needed to isolate the virus particles. First marketed by Merrell–National Laboratories.

HibVAX®. *Haemophilus influenzae* type b polysaccharide vaccine, used for routine immunization of children 24 months to 5 years of age. Launched April 1, 1986. Withdrawn from the market when ProHIBiT was licensed.

IMOGAM® Rabies. Rabies immune globulin (human) USP. Distributed by Swiftwater.

IMOVAX® Rabies. Rabies vaccine USP. Distributed by Swiftwater.

IMOVAX® Rabies I.D. Rabies vaccine USP (for preexposure). Distributed by Swiftwater.

IPOL®. Enhanced, inactivated polio vaccine, injectable. Manufactured by

Pasteur Mérieux Connaught France and distributed by Swiftwater.

JE-VAX®. Japanese encephalitis virus vaccine inactivated. Manufactured by Biken and distributed by Swiftwater.

Menomune®. Meningococcal polysaccharide vaccine, Groups A, C, Y, and W-135 combined. Used to protect against bacterial meningitis, which causes a disease of the meninges, the nerves of the lower brain in the spinal cord. Developed in Swiftwater beginning in 1971.

Mono-Vacc® (O.T.). Tuberculin skin test, old test (O.T.). Manufactured in France.

MSTA®. Mumps skin test antigen USP.

Multitest® CMI. Skin test antigens for cellular hypersensitivity. Manufactured in France.

ProHIBiT®. A conjugated polysaccharide vaccine intended for use in children to protect against *Haemophilus influenzae* type b, the leading cause of bacterial meningitis in young children. Contains the same capsular polysaccharide as HibVAX but is conjugated, or chemically bonded, to a diphtheria toxoid protein, which makes the polysaccharide more immunogenic in infants. Developed at Swiftwater in 1982 and licensed in 1987.

Tetanus toxoid. Tetanus toxoid is a clear fluid. Tetanus toxoid adsorbed is a suspension of tetanus toxoid, adsorbed (mingled) with aluminum phosphate to slow assimilation into the body and thereby enhance antibody response and immunity. It is also combined with diphtheria toxoid in two products (DT and Td) and with diphtheria and pertussis (DTaP). Used for active immunization to prevent tetanus (lockjaw), an infectious disease caused by bacteria that generally enter the body through a wound. First licensed by National Drug in 1934.

TheraCys®. Bacillus Calmette-Guerin (BCG) live (intravesical). Used in the prevention of tuberculosis, this was the first FDA-licensed BCG product for the treatment of urinary bladder cancer (carcinoma in situ). Manufactured in Canada and distributed by Swiftwater.

TriHIBit™. ActHIB, *Haemophilus* b conjugate vaccine (tetanus toxoid conjugate), reconstituted with Tripedia, diphtheria and tetanus toxoids, and acellular pertussis vaccine adsorbed. Licensed September 27, 1996, for children 15–18 months old. Infant license pending. It contains PRPT Hib conjugate from France and prevents diphtheria, tetanus, pertussis, and Hib (*Haemophilus influenzae* type b).

Tripedia®. Diphtheria and tetanus toxoids and acellular pertussis vaccine adsorbed. Licensed in 1992 for children ages 15–18 months old and in 1996 for infants. Combines traditional diphtheria and tetanus vaccines with a Japanese acellular pertussis component manufactured by the Research Foundation for Microbial Diseases of Osaka University (Biken®). Tripedia differs from whole-cell vaccines in that it contains only those parts of the pertussis bacterium that are believed to induce immunity against the disease.

Tubersol®. Tuberculin purified protein derivative (Mantoux). Manufactured in Canada.

Typhim Vi®. Typhoid fever vaccine, launched in France in 1989. Manufactured in France.

YF-VAX®. For the prevention of yellow fever. For persons 6 months and older traveling to areas where yellow fever is prevalent. Developed in the late 1940s by the Rockefeller Institute and later produced and supplied by U.S. Public Health Service, the vaccine's technology was transferred to National Drug in 1952. It is a freeze-dried product.

Appendix G

Products Licensed by the Swiftwater Laboratories

1897. Glycerinated smallpox vaccine, also called vaccine virus. Not required to be a licensed vaccine at that time.

August 1903. U.S. Treasury Department issued 12 licenses to 11 biological manufacturers. The Pocono Laboratory received license number 6, reissued on a yearly basis.

1911–12. Slee Laboratory licensed tetanus antitoxin, human. Prior to 1917, the lab produced diphtheria antitoxin; tetanus antitoxin, veterinary; antimeningitis serum; antistreptococcic serum; normal serum; vaccine serum; anticanine distemper vaccine; antityphoid vaccine typhus and paratyphoid; and antityphoid vaccine typhoid only. Gas gangrene antitoxin was produced before and during World War I. The Slees also developed a sideline of K prophylactic packets primarily for the armed forces.

1927. With the leasing of the laboratory by the National Drug Co., Arthur Slee retained the vaccine virus and marketed it under license number 6. Products bearing the National Drug Co. label were produced under license number 101.

1926. Pertussis vaccine.

January 14, 1927. Typhoid vaccine.

December 12, 1927. Diphtheria antitoxin, equine origin.

December 14, 1927. Tetanus antitoxin, equine origin.

1929. Diphtheria toxoid.

May 25, 1934. Tetanus toxoid, plain and adsorbed.

February 27, 1942. Cholera vaccine.

April 18, 1944. First commercial lot of DTP adsorbed released based on the potency of the separate components.

September 16, 1947. Influenza virus vaccine, Sharples® purified. Japanese B virus vaccine manufactured on special government contract but not licensed.

May 13, 1949. License for DTP, Ad, based on the potency of final pool.

1951. Epidemic typhus vaccine.

May 22, 1953. Yellow fever vaccine.

March 7, 1955. Tetanus and diphtheria toxoids adsorbed, for adult use.

November 15, 1961. Smallpox vaccine, freeze-dried, for domestic and government use.

April 10, 1970. Influenza virus vaccine bivalent (Fluzone®).

1967–73. Eighteen product licenses withdrawn.

July 11, 1975. Meningococcal polysaccharide vaccine, Group C.

August 18, 1975. Meningococcal polysaccharide vaccine, Group A.

December 13, 1976. Meningococcal polysaccharide vaccine, Groups A and C combined (Menomune®).

February 1, 1985. MSTA, mumps skin test antigen.

December 20, 1985. *Haemophilus* polysaccharide vaccine (HibVAX®).

June 3, 1986. *Haemophilus influenzae* type b vaccine.

December 22, 1987. *Haemophilus* conjugate vaccine, diphtheria toxoid conjugate (ProHIBiT®).

1992. Tripedia® fourth and fifth (booster) dose indication.

March 30, 1993. *Haemophilus* b conjugate vaccine (tetanus toxoid conjugate).

November 28, 1994. *Salmonella typhi* Vi capsular polysaccharide vaccine.

July 31, 1996. Tripedia for infants.

September 30, 1996. ActHIB® combined by reconstitution with Tripedia for children aged 15–18 months old (TriHIBit™).

Appendix H

Slee Family History

Marriages

Richard Child Slee to Maria Jane Orr, February 6, 1865, Bond Head, Canada. The parents of Dr. Richard Slee, the founder of the Pocono Biological Laboratories.

Dr. Richard Slee to Ella Maginnis, November 1, 1892, Swiftwater, Pennsylvania.

Arthur Maginnis Slee, son of the founder, to Phoebe Edmunds, October 9, 1915, in Lynchburg, Virginia.

Richard Edmunds Slee, grandson of the founder, to Mary Waldron Sisco, November 22, 1941, in Butler, New Jersey.

Deborah W. Slee, great-granddaughter of the founder, to Thomas Randolph Gibbs, February 17, 1968, in Charlottesville, Virginia.

Prescott Warren Slee, great-grandson of the founder, to Michele Kathleen Burnett, June 18, 1976, in Kalamazoo, Michigan.

Births

Dr. Richard Slee, the founder, September 15, 1867, in Brooklyn, New York.

Ella Maginnis Slee, wife of Dr. Richard Slee, August 30, 1870.

Elizabeth Maria Slee, sister of the founder, October 12, 1871, in South Brooklyn, New York.

Alfred Hyde Slee, brother of the founder, February 19, 1877, in Brooklyn.

Arthur Maginnis Slee, son of the founder, May 6, 1894, in Swiftwater.

Richard Edmunds Slee, son of Arthur and Phoebe and only grandson of the founder, March 29, 1917, in Brooklyn.

Deborah Waldron Slee, daughter of Richard E. and Mary Slee, July 26, 1945, in Harrisburg, Pennsylvania.

Prescott Warren Slee, son of Richard E. and Mary Slee, June 23, 1951, in Princeton, New Jersey.

Mary Carter Gibbs, daughter of Thomas R. and Deborah S. Gibbs, in Richmond, Virginia.

Katherine Waldron Slee, daughter of Prescott W. and Michele B. Slee, November 22, 1981, in Holland, Michigan.

Prescott Edmunds Slee, son of Prescott W. and Michele B. Slee, May 15, 1985, in Holland.

Deaths

Alfred Hyde Slee, 1, infant son of Richard C. and Maria J. Slee, April 14, 1878, of meningitis, 231 Schermerhorn St., Brooklyn. Brother of the founder.

Elizabeth "Lizzie" Maria Slee, 11, daughter of Richard C. and Maria J. Slee, of scarlet fever, on May 8, 1883, in Brooklyn. Sister of the founder.

Col. Arthur Maginnis, 51, father of Ella Maginnis Slee, July 10, 1891, in Swiftwater, Pennsylvania.

Richard Child Slee, 69, husband of Maria J. (Orr) Slee and father of the founder, May 1, 1912, in Swiftwater.

Maria Jane (Orr) Slee, 83, wife of Richard Child Slee, October 18, 1925.

Ella Maginnis Slee, 73, wife of Dr. Richard Slee, daughter of the late Arthur and Ella Maginnis. September 1, 1943, in Stroudsburg.

Dr. Richard Slee, 78, the founder, April 8, 1945, in Stroudsburg.

Phoebe Edmunds Slee, 78, wife of Arthur M. Slee, March 13, 1964, in Stroudsburg.

Arthur M. Slee, 74, son of the founder, December 11, 1968, in Stroudsburg.

Mary Waldron Slee, 66, wife of Richard Edmunds Slee, January 2, 1984, in Richmond.

Richard Edmunds Slee, 69, son of Arthur and Phoebe Slee, September 17, 1986, in Richmond.

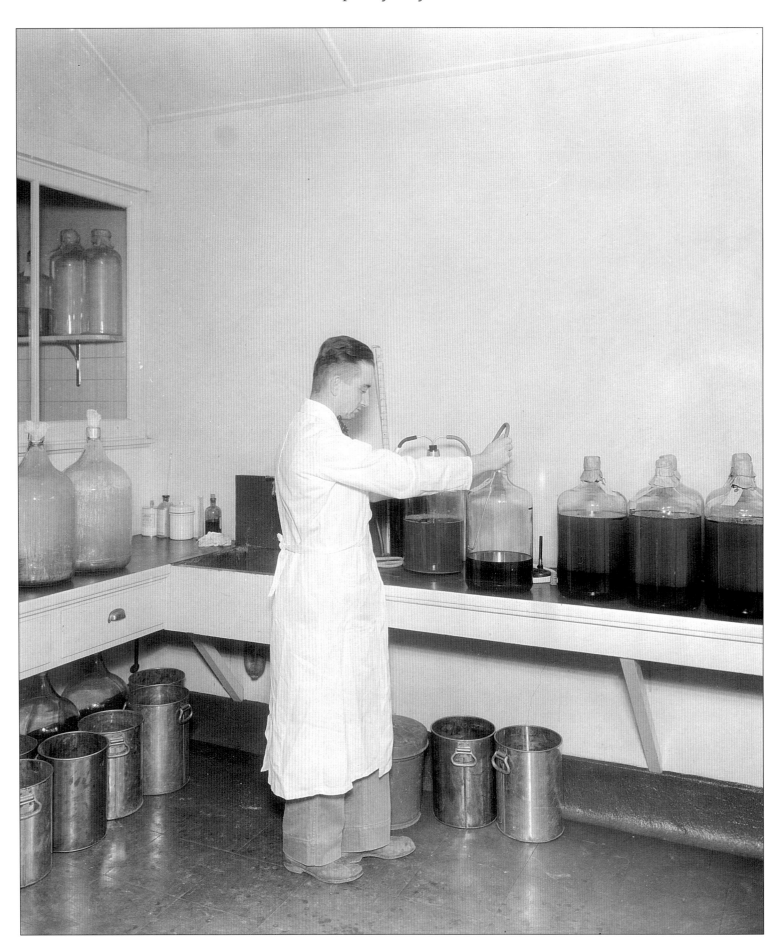

Index

Subject

Facing page: Tom McGuire collects sera by vacuum in this 1932 photo taken in Swiftwater.

Names

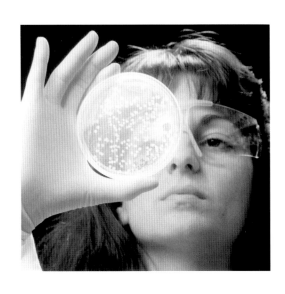

SHIRLEY LA COE	EVA MARKUS	MELISSA MURPHY	ROXANE PETERSON
JAMES LABAR	CHRISTINE MARSHALL	CHARLES MURRAY	GEOFFREY PETERSON
JON LACOMIS	MARGARET MARSHALL	LISA MURRAY	MICHAEL PETOCK
KRISTEN LADZINSKI	PAMELA MARTINEZ	ROBIN MURTHA	JOHN PETRAGLIA
DAVID LAMB	GRETA MARTOCCI	KELLY MUSCHONG	MARGARET PETRAKIS
DIANE LAMOND	EUGENE MASCOLO	LINDA MYERS	LINDA PETRO
PATRICIA LANDHEER	JAMES MATTHEWS	BRIAN MYLER	ROBERT PETRYK
BRIAN LANGAN	MICHELE MATTIOLI	GARY NABORS	BRIAN PFISTER
SYLVIA LASHER	JOSEPH MATYJEVICH	SANJAY NADKARNI	LAURA PHAIR-RUDIN
JERRY LASHLEY	JOHN MAYS	JANICE NAGELHOUT	JOHN PHILLIPS
WILLIAM LAUKAITIS	MICHAEL MAZUTIS	ROBERT NAPOLI	EDWARD PICCINI
JOSEPH LAVELLE	ANNA MC ALEAVY	VERONICA NAPOLIELLO	HILDA PICKELHAUPT
JONI LAVELLE	MARY JANE MC CAIN	MARY BETH NAUMAN	DARREN PIEPER
LEONARD LAVENDA	GEOFFREY MC CLEARY	MADELINE NEBBIA	VINCENT PIETREFESA
CLAIRE LEARN	THOMAS MC FADDEN	DOMINIQUE NERETTE	PATRICIA PIETROBON
DARREN LEBER	THOMAS MC KINNEY	WAYNE NEVELING	VENSLOUGH PILE
ANNETTE LECKSTROM	RONALD MC MASTER	CATHARINE NEWBERRY	TIMOTHY PINKOWSKI
THOMAS LEDUC	KENNETH MC MICKEN	YVONNE NEWTON	KARIN PINTERICH
CHUNG LEE	DONNA MC MICKEN	IDA NEYHART	WAYNE F PISANO
MATTHIAS LEE	PATRICK MCVERRY	DANIEL NEYHART	MARC PLATTNER
SAMSON LEE	KEVIN MC WILLIAMS	ROSELINE NOLLENBERGER	DANIEL POKRAS
WOODY LEE	DAVID MCDANIEL	ANGIE NORDMARK	SUSAN POLIZZOTTO
DIANA LEIBOLD	LAURIE MCDONALD	STEPHEN NYSTEDT	ROBERT POLIZZOTTO
ROBERT LEMMON	SEAN MCDONOUGH	FINOLA O'SULLIVAN	RUTH PONA
LINDA LESOINE	MICHAEL MCFERSON	JOSEPH OCCHIPINTI	LINDA POSSINGER
SHERRY LEWIS	BRIAN MCKENNA	JAMES ODDONO	CAROL POSTUPAK
CINDY LEWIS-KESSLER	ROBERT MCPARTLAND	THOMAS ODENWELDER	JASON PRATT
JOANN LICARI	MARYANNE MCWILLIAMS	BARBARA OPPELT	DEBORAH PRIDE
WILLIAM LIGHTBODY	CHRISTOPHER MENEELY	MONICA ORGANISCIAK	TIM PROBASCO
MARIA LISICA	CARLTON MESCHIEVITZ	MARIA ORTIZ	CHERYL PRUSS
ANTHONY LIZZA	STEVEN METZGAR	FRANCIS OSBORNE	BARBARA PRYNDA
MARIA LIZZA	MICHAEL MEYERS	MARIE OTTE	TERRIE PUMPHREY
MICHELE LOGAN	THOMAS MICKENS	JOAN OWEN	DEREK PYLE
COLLEEN LONDON	MICHELLE MICKENS	MARKUS PACE	GREGG QUATRINI
PAMELA LONG	LINDA MILASCH	VICTORIA PAGANO	JOSEPH QUINN
JOANN LOPRESTI	JOSEPH MILEY	MICHAEL PAICH	DEVRI QUINTANA
LYNETTE LORD	LORA MILLER	MICHAEL PAMUKCOGLU	MICHAEL RACKISH
JANET LORING	RAYMOND MILLER	ANTHONY PANSY	ERNEST RACZ
CHRISTOPHER LOSCALZO	HELEN MILLER	ALISON PAPAY	CYNTHIA RANSOM
JOSEPH LOUGHNEY	CAROL MITCHELL	DEBORA PARINI	MICHAELENE RAYMOND
JEFFERY LOVELACE	SUSAN MITCHELL	JAMES PARINI	DONA REBER
THOMAS LUBINSKI	MARYLOUISE MODERSKI	CHERYL PARK	KELLY REBMANN
RYAN LUKASHEFSKI	NICOLE MONICA	JIM PARKER	KATHLEEN RECTOR
THOMAS LUKE	RHONDA MONTGOMERY	KIMBERLY PARKS	RICHARD REDA
KIMBERLY LUNDQUIST	LINDA MOODY	JOHN PARRISH	ANN REED
WILLIAM LUTTMANN	LINDA MOOMAU	RONALD PASQUALE	MATTHEW REESE
MICHAEL MACEROLLO	FAITH MOORE	ARUNA PATEL	JOHN REICE
KIMBERLY MACNEILL	JACQUELINE MOORE	REECE PATTERSON	SAMUEL REID
JOHN MACRI	MAURA MORAN	VICTOR PAULUS	CYNTHIA REINHARDT
KAYLA MADISON	KATHLEEN MORGAN	DAVID PAYNTER	ALBERT REINHARDT
MARIA MAGINNIS	STEPHEN MORGAN	SHANNON PEACHER	ERICA REINHARDT
ROCK MAGNOTTA	AMY MORGAN	STEPHEN PEARCE	SUSAN REISINGER
DANIEL MAHAN	ANA MORLEY	MICHELLE PEIL	PAMELA REMEY
BEATA MALEC	DAVID MORMAK	KATHY PENDLETON	ELAINE REU
GRZEGORZ MALEC	SAMUEL MORRIS	SANDRA PENNELL	RONALD REUSSWIG
DAVID MALINZAK	LINDA MOTTS	DONALD PENSYL	RALPH REY
WENDY MANGAN	JOYCE MOYNIHAN	TIMOTHY PERDUE	DOUGLAS REYNOLDS
LOUIS MANGINO	ROBERT MRAZ	BETH PERRI	DIANE REYNOLDS
CARRIE MANNING	MATTHEW MUCHMORE	DENIS PETERS	TRACEY REZAK
LYNNE MARINUCCI	JAY MULLEN	DAROLYN PETERSON	SUZANNE REZNICEK

RYAN RIBOLDI
BRENDA RICHARDSON
SHARON RIDDICK
DENISE RIEKER
JOSEPHINE RIGGS
CHERYL RINEHART
GEORGE RINKER
DEBORAH RIOTT
R. JULIAN RITCHEY
SHEILA RIVERA
MATTHEW ROACH
STEPHEN ROBEDDA
JAMES ROBINSON
DOUGLAS ROCK
KELLY RODGERS
FREDDIE RODRIGUEZ
JOYCE ROEBER
WENDY ROEBER
JOSEPH ROGALEWICZ
BARBARA ROHL
BETTY ROLLERSON
FRED ROMANO
KATHLEEN ROSE
BARBARA ROSENBERG
FREDERICK RUBEN
ROBERT RUDZINSKI
GREGORY RUFFENACH
CANDACE RUGGIERO
JOSEPH RUIZ
CATHY RUNYON
TINA RUSS
BRENT RUTLAND
ROBERT RYALL
KELLY SAFIN
MICHAEL SALACH
DORINA SALAJAN
BRENDA SAMONY
PETER SAMONY
MARIA SANSAET
KAREN SANTONE
JOSEPH SANTONE
MARIANNE SANTORA
JOSEPH SAUKULYAK
JOHN SCALAMANDRE
JOSEPH SCARAMASTRO
ELIZABETH SCARSELLA
DOUGLAS SCHAEFER
JOHN SCHAEFFER
YVONNE SCHAEFFER
KIMBERLY SCHAFER
THOMAS SCHENKE
DAVID SCHERMERHORN
TRACY SCHIAVONE
SHERRY SCHILB
MICHAEL SCHLEGEL
CHRISTINE SCHLINK
RICHARD SCHNEIDER
JOYCE SCHOCH
TERRENCE SCHULER
SUSANNAH SCHULLER

CHERI SCOTT
CAROLYNN SCOTT
ROBERT SEAFORTH
JOANN SEALE
DALE SEBRING
ARMINDA SEESE
ROBERT SEGARRA
TED SEIDEL
KENNETH SENGHAAS
MICHAEL SEPRISH
MARK SERRA
TAMI SHAFER
KIRIT SHAH
ANTHONY SHANNON
JEFFREY SHIFF
MARK SHILLING
SHERMAN SICKLER
JAMES SIGLIN
DARYL SIMPSON
DAVID SIMS
HOWARD SIX
PATRICIA SKUDER
GREGORY SLUSAW
CARL SLUTTER
WILLEM SMIT
RICKY SMITH
LYNN SMITH
LORI SMITH
KIDREN SMITH
SANDRA SMITH
CAROLYN SMITH
MELISSA SMITH
MARLENE SMITH
STACEY SMITHLINE
TIM SNOW
JANICE SNYDER
JUDITH SOLOMONS
DANUTA SOWA
JOHN SPEER
RICHARD SPINA
MARY SPOLSKY
JENNIFER STANFORD
NANCY STAY
SHARON STEARNS
VIRGINIA STECKEL
PETER STEFURA
BETTY STEFURA
ALLEN STEIN
DORIS STELTZ
LINDA STEVENS
WENDY STEVENS
JEFFREY STEWART
JASON STEWART
CYNTHIA STINSON
MICHAEL STIRR
ROBERT STOBACK
DAVID STONE
JUDITH STOUT
MICHELLE STRUSS
CAROL STURIALE

LAUREEN SULLIVAN
JEROME SULZER
LORETTA SURLS
SUZANNE SUSTER
DIRK SUTHERLAND
RACHELLE SUTTON
CHRISTOPHER SWAIN
KATHY SWAN
SHARON SYLVESTER
WENDY TALBOTT
JAMES TAYLOR
LOIS TAYLOR
HOLLY TAYLOR
BETHANY TEMPEL
LEE TERMINI
SANTIAGO TEXEIRA
JEANNE THALLMAYER
JENNIFER THOMAS
SARAH THOMPSON
CARMEN THOMPSON
CARA THOMPSON
THOMAS THORN
DIANNE THORN
DOROTHY THORPE
LESLIE TICE
KARI TIERNEY
BRUCE TILLEY
MARK TINSLEY
ERIC TISCHLER
TIMOTHY TOLAN
EDWARD TOMPKINS
RONALD TONKYRO
TRACY TOVO
JOSEPH TRANSUE
RICHARD TROIANI
PIERRE TROTEMANN
DONNA TROTT
FRANK TULL
CYNTHIA TURZINSKI
ALAN TYSON
EDWARD UTTER
CYNTHIA VANDERWEEL
LYNNAE VELDHUIZEN
EMMANUEL VIDOR
DANIEL VITANZA
H. THOMAS VOIGE
JANET VOORHEES
FLETCHER VOORHEES
RALPH VOSDINGH
KELLY WALL
DONNA WALLER
DOLORES WALSH
LEANN WALTERS
RODNEY WALTZ
DONALD WARAKOMSKI
JAMES WARAKOMSKI
WILLIAM WARKE
KERRI WARNER
WILLIAM WARNER
BRIDGETTE WASHINGTON

MICHAEL WATSON
DIANA WATTS
JOHN WATTS
DEAN WEHR
HEATHER WEHRMEISTER
LESTER WEINMAN
LINNEA WEINMAN
KAREN WERKHEISER
LARRY WERKHEISER
THOMAS WESCOTT
JAMES WESTBROOK
GARY WESTRACK
CHARLES WHITAKER
ALAN WHITAKER
EDWARD WHITE
JOHN WHITE
HEATHER WHITESELL
MATTHEW WILCOX
DAVID WILLIAMS
LINDA WILLIAMS
JIMMY WILLIAMS
ROBIN WILLIAMS
MARCIA WILLIAMS
ANGELA WILSON
LEESA WILSON
JOSHUA WILSON
ROBERT WOLF
CARINA WOODRICH
KELLY WOODS
WALTER WOODS JR.
WILLIAM WOODWORTH
DARCY WRIGHT
LOUIS WRIGHT
XINGHAO WU
STANLEY WYSOCKY
MICHAEL YACUBOSKI
PATRICIA YANAVAGE
WENDY YOLINSKY
DOMINICK YORK
DENISE YOUNG
MARY ZABINSKI
SUSAN ZABRISKIE
JOHN ZAHRADNIK
DORIS ZAJAC
ANGELA ZEGLIN